Herbal Medication

Written by Peter Dunn

Contents

The medical information and advice in this book are based upon the experience and research of the author. Persons using this book should consult an appropriate health care provider when questions of medical treatment and care arise. The author assumes no responsibility and is not liable for adverse effects resulting from the use of any advice or information contained in this book.

Chapter One

What is Herbal Medicine?

Herbal medicine is the oldest and most popular form of healing in the world but it continues to defy our conventional understanding of medicine. It has no inventor, no country or culture owns it, and it has no known starting point in history. This sets it apart from all other forms of medicine or healing. It is also a universal medicine. There is no recorded civilization or culture, across the world or through history that has not used plants for medicine. Eighty per cent of the world's population still relies on plant medicines. There is even evidence that our prehistoric human ancestors used plant medicines and that wild animal's still do. Plants are -as natural as water, breathing or sunrises. They lay good claim to being the only natural medicine and are as useful today as they ever were.

But what is herbal medicine? What makes it so different and so universal? The simplest definition is 'the use of plant material as medicine'. For many people, this includes using whole plants, making simple extracts like teas, and the extraction and purification of single ingredients of plants to make modern pharmaceutical drugs like digoxin or morphine. Other people exclude the extraction of single ingredients because, they argue, the natural mixture of chemicals in plants is what makes them so effective and safe (see Chapter 6).

This simplistic definition is inadequate. Throughout history and particularly in modern herbal medicine, how the plants were used has been essential to the practice of herbal medicine. The herbs have been used within distinct systems of medicine. Each system is identified by its own philosophy of health, a theory of disease causation, and a clear logic and method in using the herbs as treatment.

In contrast with the system of homoeopathy, for example, which was defined precisely by its inventor, there are several different systems of herbal medicine in use today. Throughout history there have been many more. Any attempt to identify herbal medicine with a single system is therefore not only inappropriate, but might deprive us of valuable insight into the mysteries of healing with plants. All of the history of herbal medicine contributes to present knowledge. It was Hippocrates who described medicine as more an art than a science, and any art is best appreciated by reflection, not definition.

The filtering of herbal medicine through thousands of years of practice in different countries and cultures has produced many different approaches and philosophies. Far from being conflicting approaches they are, like different literary traditions, products of the intellectual and physical resources of the time and often astound by their creativity. Many ancient beliefs about both healing and herbs have been shown to be correct by modern science. Before describing modern herbal medicine, it is helpful to reflect on how the history and universality of herbal medicines have influenced current practice.

Plants as Medicine and Food

Our dependence on plants is remarkable. Despite human mastery over technology, we cannot create our own food. Human survival in the most advanced societies is totally dependent on cultivating plants and animals in a manner not fundamentally different from hunter-farmers 20,000 years ago.

The method of cultivation has improved but farmers still sow seeds and harvest plants, or grow plants to feed to animals which are also harvested. Of course, the food industry makes products from mayonnaise to muesli but what are these but modified plant products from farms? There is no clear boundary between plants as food and as medicine. Both are used to keep our bodies performing properly.

Food supplies nutrients which are essential for health. For example, without Vitamin C, bones and connective tissue do not grow or function properly. It protects against damage from chemicals called- free radicals, which can cause cancer. It stimulates the body's own production of the chemical cortisol, a natural steroid that is essential to life and which is used as a drug in many illnesses. Dietary iron is essential for healthy blood, without which oxygen cannot be absorbed from air in the lungs and the body's vital chemical processes slowdown or stop.

Food must also contain enough indigestible material (roughage or fibre) to stop constipation; if there is insufficient fibre, both absorption of nutrients from food and excretion of waste materials will stop and we become unhealthy.

Plant medicines also stimulate the body's processes. Bitter herbs like gentian *(Gentiana lutea)* stimulate the release of digestive juices in the stomach and intestine. Liquorice *(Glycyrrhiza glabra)* stimulates the adrenal gland to produce cortisol, which helps the body fight diseases like rheumatism and psoriasis. Herbs like ginger *(Zingiber officinale)* and chilli *(CapsicUm minimum)* stimulate the circulation of blood. There are many plants with antimicrobial and antiseptic properties because they contain chemicals which kill microbes; other plants, like
Echinacea angustijolia, stimulate the body's immune system, which helps to defeat microbial infections.

As food or medicine, many plants often work in similar ways to protect or promote health. The old saying, 'an apple a day keeps the doctor away' -shows ancestral wisdom in the value of plants. How it was discovered which plants were edible and nutritious invites fascinating speculation. The term 'trial and error' is the easiest explanation. The most important choice was between safe and toxic plants. Safe plants may be more or less nutritious and many food plants, even today, are eaten more for pleasure than nutritional value. Foods like cucumber and cauliflower have no significant nutritional value but are eaten for texture or flavour. Samuel Johnson didn't like anything about cucumber. He said it should be 'well sliced, and dressed with pepper and vinegar, and then thrown out as good for nothing'. Our diet is made up of many foods, few of which are individually essential for life, but in total they supply enough of the essential nutrients. Choosing medicinal plants must have required different skills. Whereas food plants were chosen more for their availability and taste with only the most general association with health, plant medicines must have been chosen for specific illnesses at specific times. The choice had to be more critical, more accurate, and more certain because specific effects were sought at specific times.

Imagine you are living 5,000 years ago. You and your fellow pioneers live among lush lowlands with rivers and open grasslands spread beneath wooded hills offering many varieties of trees hanging with berries and fruits. It is possible to picture how you might discover a plant to wrap around a wound to stop bleeding. The application of the plant and the stopping of the bleeding would have happened within minutes of each other.

Cause and effect could be seen. Plants rich in tannins, like tormentil *(Potentilla erecta)* or witch hazel *(Hamamelis virginiana)*, would have stood out because of their rapid effect in stopping bleeding.

But how were plant medicines that changed the menstrual cycle, purified the blood, hastened the healing of broken bones, or expelled kidney stones identified? The herbs used for these conditions work over weeks or months. You might have chosen a plant to try against pain in the loin caused by kidney stones.

How would you have worked out whether your test plant rather than any of the many plants you were eating daily as food had any positive result you observed? The longer the medicine took to work, the more you would have been exposed to additional factors that would have made it difficult to identify the healing plant. All this testing was done with only memory to record your results and without the luxury of a local library in which to check what other people had discovered.

The mysteries of discovering plant medicines are still observed. Researchers in Africa who spent thirty years watching chimps often noticed that one group of daisy-like plants, *Aspilia,* was eaten only occasionally compared to food leaves. They also noticed that its leaves were eaten in a totally different manner to the eating of food plants. The *Aspt1ia* leaves were carefully selected, one at a time, instead of grabbing bunches of food leaves, and the leaf was put into the mouth and carefully rolled around before being swallowed whole. At first the observers thought the *Aspilia* was simply a stimulant but when they tasted the plant, they found it was so bitter that not even chimps could be expected to eat it for pleasure alone!

Almost by chance, the researchers met some anthropologists who were working with the local Tongwe people and discovered that the *Aspilia* was one of the most used herbal medicines in East Africa. It was made into a tea to treat wounds and burns, but especially for stomach upsets and intestinal worms. It was then noticed that the chimps and the local people choose *the same three species* of *Aspilia* and ignored others.

Further checking of years of accumulated notes on chimp behaviour led to more discoveries. Chimps appeared to use other plant medicines. One chimp ate leaves of *Lippea* and then found a peaceful spot where she lay quietly. Local people used the same species to treat stomach ache. Later chimps with diarrhoea were seen to choose a plant which local people used to treat diarrhoea caused by intestinal parasites. Examination of the chimps droppings showed high populations of parasites.

Other species like the fig tree, *Ficus exasperata,* or the latex-rich plant *Commelina* are also known to be used against infections by both people and chimps.

The researchers had to send plant samples to sophisticated laboratories for chemical analysis which confirmed that these plants contained chemicals that kill bacteria, fungi and worms.

Some even have chemicals which stimulate the immune system to protect from parasitic infection. While scientists are excited with their potential new drugs for humans, we should meditate on how the Tongwe and the chimps discovered them at all.

Finding plant medicines is remarkable enough but there is evidence that the same, or closely related plants, were used for the same conditions in different corners of the globe without any communication being possible. The Australian Aborigine was using a relative of the Jamaican Sarsaparilla plant for the same tonic and alterative purposes 40,000 years ago. The Sarsaparilla genus, *Smilax,* is also found in use in South American and Indian medicine. The Aborigines not only discovered the narcotic alkaloids of *Nicotiaruz,* the tobacco plant, for themselves, but also were found chewing small balls of it 'when the white settlers arrived. Liquorice has been used for over 2,000 years and related species are known to have been used around the

Euphrates River, in Russia and in China. Its ancient uses were similar wherever it has been used and its benefits as an expectorant, demulcent and adrenal stimulant because of its steroidal-like action. Ginger species are common to most recorded uses of plants. It has been cultivated for so long that no one is sure what the original wild parent was or where it came from. One species of *Hibiscus* has been used to regulate fertility in many countries from the Caribbean to the Pacific Ocean, including Thailand on the way.

Although it offers a convenient explanation, there is no way of knowing the part intuition played in identifying medicinal plants by animals or humans. Unless intuition is the same process in all species, it hardly explains how some medicines were put to the same uses in different parts of the world. The discovery of over 2,000 plant medicines also suggests that there is something very special about plants and our relationship with them throughout evolution and history. Believers in some form of God accept that the plants were created for our use, whether as food, fuel, shelter, clothing or medicine. But evolutionists may argue with equal conviction that the evolution of humans and other animals progressed with such intimate connection with plants that we are biologically one large organism. This notion runs close to Lovelock's Gaia hypothesis. He sees the earth, its atmosphere and everything living on it as one interconnected living energy system and being. All things work together towards balance or homoeostasis. That plants give us the nutrients to grow and reproduce as well as the medicines to cure our diseases could be seen as elementary to the Gaia explanation.

Whatever explanation you choose, all our knowledge about the medicinal value of plants shows that they are profoundly valuable. To ignore them is to deny natural laws. To reject them is to waste a prime natural resource.

Of Myths and Magic

Since herbal medicine has been in use since the beginnings
of civilization, it is not surprising that the power of herbs has
been associated with mystical or superstitious beliefs. People
explained their world using their limited resources for
observation and understanding natural phenomena.
Remember that it was only with the invention of the
microscope in the seventeenth century that it was possible to
see the bacteria that caused infectious diseases and to dispel
the notions that evil spirits and demons caused illness.
The Doctrine of Signatures, which was put about by the
16thcentury physician Paracelsus, is one example of myth. It
must have been convincing, for it dominated thinking for
nearly 400 years. The Doctrine said that God had given us
herbs and had endowed each useful plant with visible signals
to guide our selection. Thus yellow dock was for jaundice
because it was yellow. Likewise lungwort was good for lung
disease because its leaves resembled human lungs; walnuts
were head-shaped and so were good for headaches; henbane
was destined for tooth aches because its seed pod looked like
a tooth. The
Doctrine looks very unconvincing today but in its time it was
more than plausible. Not only was there no science to offer
other explanations but the church, learned physicians and
religion were generally more socially influential than today.
It is a mistake, however, to believe that everyone accepted
glibly such imaginative attempts to explain the world. In
1597, the famous English herbalist John Gerard made a
loose and entertaining translation of a Dutch Herbal written
by Dodoen in 1583. Gerard could not help himself from
pointing out what he considered to be farcical attributes of
plants. For example, the mandrake plant has long been
linked to magic - it was supposed to be human-shaped and
utter a scream as it was pulled from the ground - but Gerard
said of these beliefs:

"There have been many ridiculous tales brought up of this plant, whether of old wives, or some runnagate Surgeons of Physicke-mongers I know not, (a title bad enough for them) but sure someone or more that sought to make themselves famous and skilful above others, were the first brochers of that error I speak of. They added further, That it is never or very seldom to be found growing but under a gallows, where the matter that hath fallen from the dead body hath given it the shape of a man; and the matter of a woman, the substance of a female plant; with many other such doltish dreames. They fable further and affirm, That he who would take up a plant thereof must tie a dog thereunto to pull it up, which will give a great shreeke at the digging up; otherwise if a man should do it, he would surely die is short space thereafter. All which dreames and old wives tales you shall from henceforth cast out of your books and memory; knowing this, that they are all and every part of them false and most untrue: for I myself and my servants also have digged up, planted, and replanted very many, and yet never could either perceive shape of man or woman ...

The magic of mandrake and many of the more drastic magical properties of the plants are thought to have arisen to protect the formulae of medicines used by physicians or herb women. In the days before patent laws protected inventors' rights, it-was a necessary business skill to put the fear of death into any patient who might want to harvest their own medicinal plants. The more horrific the consequences, the less likely the lay person was to make their own medicine and the higher your status was as a healer for having the special knowledge and skill to handle such powerful plants."

Often the myths were derived from the need for hope to triumph over the fear of uncertainty. Simple myths like the carrying of plants as good luck charms were very common. The roots of common plantain known as lamb's tongue *(Plantago major)* used to be hung about the neck to dispel grief or ward off diseases. Gerard condemned such notions as 'ridiculous toyes.' Mugwort *(Artemisia vulgaris)* had been used as a charm since the days of Pliny. A piece tied about a traveller's clothing was said to be protective not only against tiredness but also against any poisonous medicine and even wild beasts. Of course, valid medicinal uses often lay behind the myths. Both mugwort and plantain are valuable remedies in modern herbal medicine.

Perhaps it is more extraordinary that similar myths continue to exist today. Bring hawthorn flowers into the house and many people believe that a family death will soon follow. Many people still believe that you must ask permission of an elder tree before picking the flowers or berries for fear of risking-angering the witches that live therein.

In the midlands of England mistletoe is left on apple trees for good luck even though it harms the trees.

Sometimes plant medicines are still associated with witches and spells. Sadly, this is based on a set of mistaken ideas. Power, religion and ritual have always been closely linked. Usually the priests were men and rituals were often used to create mystery and allegiance. Hallucinogenic drugs and narcotic herbs were used regularly to create spiritualistic trance-like states in which there was dancing and chanting. That is the origin of the cliché image of witches dancing around steaming cauldrons containing eye of newt, toadstools and bat wings. The witches of the middle ages were women, usually herb women who gathered local herbs and made healing remedies or potions for the sick. They were undercutting the male physicians and irritated the male priests who also dabbled in healing. The result was a smear campaign and thousands of innocent women healers were drowned or burned at the stake to protect the monopoly interests of powerful men.

All too often the sinister aspects of magic were exaggerated.

Paracelsus believed in magic. He wasn't thinking of witches' spells but 'the magical powers of the soul of man ... and I will tell you that only he who has acquired this power can be a true physician. If our physicians did possess it, their books might be burnt and their medicines thrown into the ocean, and the world would be all the better for it.' This magic was nothing more than 'strong faith in omnipotent power of all good, that can accomplish everything if it acts through a human mind that is in harmony with it'. This required faith, prayer and imagination. Examples of the same form of magic are found in the ceremonies of Christianity and other religions or the world 'today

Most of the myths and magic reflect the importance of plants in daily life.

Old Wives' Tales and Folklore

Women have always been associated with herbal remedies and healing. Not only were they collectors of herbs for the apothecaries in the towns, they were herbalists in their own right and are an important part of the healing heritage. In the middle ages, women were the household healers. They collected the local herbs, prepared the remedies and administered to the sick. They weren't formally trained, but often provided the only available medicine. As recently as last century, doctors were an elite group who concentrated their services in the towns and cities and whose fees kept the poor from their doors.

It is a mistake to assume that the doctors had safe and effective medicine while the women's medicines were useless fancy. Some argue that the poor were better off without the physicians. In 1685 Charles II died. He died a horrific death at the hands of his physicians, who we can assume fairly must have been the best in the land. Christine Stockwell in her book, *Nature's Pharmacy,* on the history of natural medicines chronicled his treatment thus:

On 2 February, while being shaved, the king was seized with a convulsion and collapsed, probably with a blood clot. First he was bled. An enema and two purgatives were administered, followed by an enema containing mallow leaves, violets, beetroot, camomile, fennel, linseed, cinnamon, cardamom, saffron and aloes - among other things. He was given a snuff of powdered hellebore and another of cowslips. He was given, to drink, a mixture of barley water, liquorice and sweet almond draughts of white wine, a cocktail of absinthe and anise and extracts of thistle leaves, mint, rue, angelica. Internal treatment continued with slippery elm, peony, lavender, lime flowers, lily of the valley, melon seeds and dissolved pearls. The physicians carried on their unholy assault with gentian root, nutmeg, quinine and cloves. They shaved the king's head and rubbed in powdered blistering beetles, meanwhile applying a drawing plaster of Burgundy pitch and pigeon droppings to his feet. They brought in the Bezoar stones - perhaps thinking that he had been poisoned. None of this improved the king's condition even though a special dose of Raleigh's antidote was forced down his throat and, after four days, during which he apologized for taking such 'an unconscionable time a-dying', the king died, surely with a sigh of relief.

The label 'old wives' is a dismissive term for women healers and the 'tales' are their plant remedies. Many such remedies have been passed down the generations for centuries and have been confirmed by recent research. Far from being a parlour joke, the old wives' tales represent possibly the most exhausting and demanding testing process that has ever been conducted for any medicine.

For centuries women were responsible for treating the members of their household. Sometimes one or more women in the local community would be recognized as particularly skilled.

Few people could read or write, so the information was passed from mother to daughter down the generations. Women's work was demanding of time and energy. The choice of herbal medicines and the sieving of information to pass on would have come under the strongest selection pressure. It is difficult to imagine that useless herbs would have survived long. There was no time to waste on harvesting, storing and preparing remedies from plants that simply did not work.

Each household and each community was in effect a very practical laboratory. Each remedy was put through thousands of experiments each year, the information gathered and compared by the researching 'old wives', and passed on to the next generation. Each remedy was put through a continuous testing process, year after year. Each year there were different researchers and also an increasing pool of information with which to evaluate the herbs. It is not surprising that many ancient remedies are still in use today, even though science has still not discovered why most of them should work.

The accumulated result is a list of medicinal herbs and a great body of knowledge and experience about their use. This is folklore and it is worth questioning the motives of anybody who dismisses its value. Many folkloric uses of herbs have led to important medicines being discovered. Aspirin, the most widely-used painkiller in the world, was discovered by a German chemist who analyzed the ingredients of the meadowsweet, which had been a popular remedy for rheumatic pains for centuries. The drug Aspirin is a synthetic version of the natural salicylic acid and is named after the original name of meadowsweet, *Spirea ulmana*. The most famous heart drug, digoxin, was discovered only because an English doctor looked into the ingredients of an old folk remedy used by a local woman to cure patients of the dropsy (an old term for accumulation of fluid in the tissues) when doctors had failed.

The folk remedy contained leaves of the foxglove *(Digitalis purpurea)* from which digoxin was and still is prepared.

The herbs found in folklore are a combination of local and imported herbs. New herbs were introduced initially through invasion. The Romans brought garlic, celandine, parsley, coriander, mustard, onions, rosemary and nettles to Britain in their medicine kits. World trade brought more herbs and spices from around the world, Ginger, cinnamon, chili, and rosemary are all herbs brought to Britain originally for culinary use, but each was used as medicine in its country of origin. When Europeans settled in North America, they discovered the native

Americans' herbal medicines began using them and brought them back to Europe. In the practice of modern herbal medicine at least a dozen of North American herbs are regularly used.

Medicinal herbs like cinchona from South America, ginseng from China, hydrastis from North America, and Melaleuca (or Tea tree) from Australia, have entered herbalists' dispensaries around the world.

This international folklore contains not only a list of valuable healing plants, but a wide and variable knowledge about the nature of disease, its treatment and health. Since the information about disease and healing has been drawn from so many cultures and times, it is no surprise that many of the explanations of disease are not universally accepted. The average Western doctor doesn't explain illness in terms of liver fire and Chi meridians as a Chinese doctor might. However, both doctors claim to treat their patients successfully. The theatrical dance ceremonies and calls to the Gods to remove evil spirits from the sick in some forms of traditional African medicines are little more than the same placebo devices which are used in Western medicine. The dances help convince the patient that healing will work, just as it has been shown that a tablet of pure sugar acts as a tranquillizer in Britain so long as it is obtained in exchange for a doctor's prescription and is coloured blue!

There is no one folklore but a continuous body of knowledge being exchanged within the community, between communities, and between cultures and countries. At each step, something is learned and something is shared. Local folklore is always a careful selection of the most available plants, the most relevant theories of disease and treatment, and the most effective remedies from this moving mass of knowledge.

Folklore is the root of modern herbal medicine. It explains how the list of nearly 2,000 medicinal plants has accumulated and why there is no single approach to using herbs.

Modern Medical Herbalism

Despite the many different ways of using herbs around the world during the last 3,000 years or so, the main forms of herbal medicine in today's world are based on two main schools of thought: the energetic principles first seen in Hippocrates' writings and modern scientific herbal medicine. Most practicing herbalists use elements of both.

THE ENERGETIC PRINCIPLES OF HEALING

The Greeks, especially under Hippocrates, started developing the first non-magical theories of disease and health. Hippocrates is claimed as the father of modern medicine mainly for his scientific approach to observing the patient and taking a detailed history before making the diagnosis. But his .theories of disease centred on his rather basic concepts of physiology. He considered that the human body was made up of four humours - blood, phlegm, yellow bile and black bile - and that these things 'make up its constitution and cause its pains and health'.

He didn't leave a clear definition of the humours but said that 'common usage has assigned to them specific and different names because there are essential differences in their appearance.

Phlegm is not like blood, nor is blood like bile, nor bile like phlegm. Indeed how could they be alike when there is no similarity of appearance and when they are different to the sense of touch?' His humours were based on different substances which could be coughed or vomited and on the well-known substance that flowed from a cut or wound.

The most important point about the four humours was how they explained disease, not how they match current understanding of anatomy or physiology. Hippocrates said health would follow 'whenever the four humours are in the correct proportion to each other, both in strength, and are well mixed'.

This is the beginning of the concept of holistic healing, which focuses on balance or harmony among all functions of the body.

Other common terms that reflect the same sense of balance are homoeostasis or equilibrium. Chinese, Ayurvedic (Indian) and Unani systems of healing are based on these concepts of balance.

Herbal medicine, homoeopathy and acupuncture are also concerned with identifying and correcting imbalances.

The Greeks identified four elements which influenced the body - earth, air, fire and water - and related these to measures of energy they called cold, dry, hot or moist. The same five elements are seen in Chinese and Ayurvedic medicine. Energy was essential to the balance in the body and while it was always present to some degree, its flow in and out of the body and between parts of the body were essential to health and disease.

Even medicines were classified according to their energy as hot or cold, an idea which is still widespread in traditional medicines throughout the world.

The herbal medicine used by the native North Americans made an impact on the white settlers from Europe in the eighteenth century. Not only did they have the medicinally useful native plants of North America to draw on, they also used heat and steam treatments to cure the sick. One white settler, Samuel Thomson, became variously infamous and famous with his ideas on healing. He believed that cold was the cause of most disease and saw that cold was little more than a shortage of body heat. His treatments relied on steam baths and heating herbs like cayenne and the local herb lobelia *(Lobelia iriflata)*. Lobelia is a powerful emetic which Thomson used to rid the body of toxins. His approach brought ridicule from the physicians who were using poisons like calomel (mercury) and drastic bleeding, even though Thomson's patients got well while those of the physicians died in agony.

Thomson admitted two influences on his ideas. One was an old woman herb-gatherer who taught him the local roots she used to make hot teas that made her patients sweat. The other was the. Hippocratic notion of energy and balance that he learned from reading the original texts by the 'father of the healing arts'.

Thomson's ideas were modified by the late nineteenth century to the vital force theories of the group of herbalists who were known as the physiomedicalists. These herbalists also followed theories of energy and balance, but concentrated more on the role of the nervous system as a regulator of balance and hence health. They tended to use more herbs that would relax or stimulate the various tissues or organs of the body.

Modern Western medicine does not and never really did embrace the same notions. The Hippocratic insistence on detailed observation of illness and history taking have been adopted but his notions of balance have no place in the theory and practice of Western orthodox medicine. Rather, it developed along a slightly more pragmatic line, which saw the body as a collection of physical organs and functions, anyone of which might break down like a part in a car or clock. If a car's brakes wear out every six months they are duly replaced.

Never mind that the driver might accelerate too quickly and drive too fast, both of which require excessive stamping on the brake pedal. The same car probably uses petrol inefficiently, wears tires quickly, burns out the clutch and has gearbox damage. A Hippocratic mechanic would be concerned with all the points of wear and tear on the car and would want (even though manners might prohibit it) to raise the matter of driving technique with the owner of the car. Perhaps treatment of the driver might improve the health of both person and vehicle.

This focus of Western medicine only on the parts of the body that are diseased is also known as reductionism. This means reducing the problem of a malfunctioning body down to a list of its parts, which are looked at one at a time, in isolation from the whole body. Reductionist medicine is designed to ignore the whole of an ill patient and is the opposite of holism. The· differences in philosophy between these two ways of seeing the patient are so great that it is usually very difficult for a doctor trained in reductionist medicine to begin to think holistically.

MODERN SCIENTIFIC HERBALISM

Modern scientific herbalism, represents efforts to understand the herbal remedies. Advances in biochemistry have allowed better insight into the chemical constituents of plants. Most plants contain thousands of chemicals, many of which have been identified as the active ingredients in herbal remedies. Combinations of active ingredients help explain the long established combination of actions in single herbs. Meadowsweet *(Filipendula ulmaria)* , for example, contains methyl salicylate, tannins and flavonoids, which help explain its actions as anti-inflammatory, astringent, and mild pain-reliever. Scientific herbalists can choose herbs for their known ingredients and actions, as well as for their traditional uses, which are often explained partially, if not totally, by their known active ingredients.

Pharmacology, which is the study of how drugs work as medicine, and clinical studies of herbal medicines have increased understanding of herbs. Garlic has been used for centuries to 'thin the blood'. Researchers in Germany discovered in 1980that eating cloves of garlic daily reduces blood cholesterol and decreases the stickiness of platelet cells in the blood, both of which 'thin the blood' and help prevent heart disease. Feverfew has a long traditional use as a reliever of headaches, especially migraines. A clinical trial in London proved this correct and also showed that eating a few leaves daily could prevent migraines as well as help stop a migraine attack.

Chemistry and pharmacology provide valuable confirmation of traditional knowledge, but cannot yet explain everything that is already known about herbs. Many plants have measurable health effects that cannot be accounted for by their known chemistry; herbs often also produce a greater healing response than could be predicted by the known amounts of their ingredients. It is often shown that such responses are due to the particular combinations of natural ingredients rather than to any single chemical. The action of the whole plant is greater than the sum of its parts, which is one good reason why herbalists still prefer using whole plants than single chemicals extracted from them.

Modem herbalists combine the concepts of energy balance with traditional experience of herbs, tempered by the latest scientific findings about the content and actions of plant medicines. They are holistic practitioners who use theories of health and herbal treatments that had their origins thousands of years ago but also incorporate current ideas where relevant to 'fine tune' their skills.

This vast and varied pool of knowledge and experience makes modem herbal medicine an eclectic profession rich in variety.

Around the core of holism, concern with energy and balance, and the use of whole plant treatments, differences in emphasis or tradition can be found. Some practitioners stick religiously to the use of whole plant remedies, whereas others may also use some isolated plant extracts. Many use Western medical approaches to the definition of disease but search for causes in the energy and balance of the whole person. Others may incorporate elements of the Chinese or Ayurvedic definitions of disease and their approaches to diagnosis and treatment. Although European herbalists already use herbs from all over the world, there is growing interest in Chinese herbs and some practitioners may use more of these than others.

The more effort given to defining herbal medicine, the more elusive its unique character and the greater the dispute about its contribution to human health. To say it is 'the use of plants as medicine' has the appeal of simplicity but is inadequate and misleading. The beliefs, or philosophy, about health and illness are as important as the use of herbs as medicine. Throughout the world there are many such beliefs and hence many approaches to herbal medicine. Rather than attempting to tie down herbal medicine with a definition, it is more useful to appreciate its evolution and diversity, through which the unique essence of herbal medicine can be best understood.

Chapter Two

The History of Herbal Medicine

All history is limited by the records left behind. This obvious fact means that our knowledge of plant medicines in past centuries is largely restricted to written records. Much of the use of herbs was, and continues to be, common to the poorer groups in society. Since the poor tend to be the least literate, we know very little of their daily lives and hence their experience of herbal medicines. We can only dream of the information lost as the thousands of women herb gatherers died. Even today we are losing the unwritten wisdom of our grandparents as the last generation to use herbal medicines regularly in the home. The majority of available records are from the wealthier and more educated ends of society but they still convey a fascinating pedigree for today's herbal legacy.

The earliest evidence of plant medicines comes not from written records but from pre-human debris in an isolated mountain cave. In 1951, Kurdish farmers directed an American anthropologist to a cave in the Zagros Mountains of Iraq. The floor of the cave, known as Shindar, contained the remains of a 60,000 year old Neanderthal burial site. Among the bones were the fragments of plants bound in the form of a wreath. This was no ordinary wreath; for it contained seven rather dull looking plants instead of colourful flowers. All seven of them are known today for their medicinal properties: cornflower, yarrow, groundsel, grape hyacinth, hollyhock, ephedra, and St Barnaby's thistle.

Opium poppy seeds *(Papaver somniferum)* were found in more recent Bronze and Copper Age remains of settlements on lake shores in Switzerland. The narcotic effects of poppy resin are so easily experienced by anyone with access to fresh plants, it is inconceivable that the poppies were not grown for their stupefying effects. The opium poppy is cursed today for the narcotic effects of its sap derivative, heroin, but it must not be forgotten that the same sap is also the source of one of the most used and most valuable pain relievers, morphine.

The claim for oldest written record goes to the Chinese emperor, Shen Nung, who wrote his *Great Herbal* somewhere between 3,000 and 2,700 BC. This remarkable book contained 365 medicinal plants, including many which are still used, and it remains in print to this day. So great was Shen Nung's impact on Chinese medicine that he is known as the father of Chinese medicine. Herbs have remained a major part of traditional Chinese medicine and they have produced the most continuous set of records in the world on the use and evaluation of herbal medicines.

The origins of Western herbalism are found in the Biblical lands of the Sumerians, between the Euphrates and Tigris rivers. Thanks to their invention of writing and preference for scratching information into wet clay tablets, their early herbals survived burial in the rubble of decaying cities. Their oldest surviving tablets date from around 2,500 BC and list over 1,000 plants, which is impressive for a region known for its deserts.

More recent Assyrian clay tablets from the personal library of King Ashurbanipal in around 650 BC list over 250 herbal medicines. These included dates, figs, anise, juniper berries, coriander, caraway, willow, and the two flowering plants oleander and jasmine.

The Egyptians left behind a vast amount of information about their medicinal habits. Much of this information was found in the personal museums, or tombs, of their leaders. Well preserved specimens of foods, medicines and other essential travelling resources were buried with their pharaohs and other notables. We must thank, if that is the right word, the Egyptians for remedies like castor oil and opium. Their most interesting record is the Ebers papyrus. This seventy-foot long parchment scroll dating from 1500BC revealed not only the names of herbs but also prescriptions for their use in named diseases. Isis, the Egyptian goddess who was said to hold all medicinal knowledge in her power, and who transmitted it to the healers, has left her mark on Western doctors. Her symbolic staff with an entwined snake, which was reputed to seek out medicinal herbs, is still used as the symbol of modern doctors. Not only was Isis a woman, but her medicine was largely herbal.

The Bible is an interesting historical record of medicine. Over 40 plant medicines are listed. Frankincense and myrrh were so valued that they were carried across the desert by the three wise men as a birthday present to the infant Christ; These are the pungent resins that exude from the bark of two trees that grow in the hot, dry deserts of the Middle East. Frankincense is used nowadays mainly in church incense, but myrrh is still used as a powerful antiseptic. Other Biblical herbs include Balm of Giliad, wormwood (Artemisia absinthium), aloes, camphor, nettles, and ginseng as well as such common household items as figs, garlic, cumin, cinnamon, mustard, hyssop and juniper.

Any traveler to the remote villages and islands of Greece who wanders around the back streets where open markets are held will experience an ancient herbal tradition that began in Greece. Country peasants will be found selling bunches and bags of medicinal herbs gathered from the hills. As early as 1500 BC in Greece, wanderers known as rhizotomists gathered herbs to sell to healers like the famous Aesculapius. He was said to be the son of Apollo and had a daughter called Hygieia, from whose name comes the word 'hygiene'. The Hippocratic Oath, which modem doctors swear to uphold, promises allegiance to Aesculapius as well as to Hippocrates.

Hippocrates not only set standards for the practice of modem medicine, he also used herbs, many of which are still in use. His medicine chest contained almonds, anise, basil, burdock, cabbage, cardamom, cloves, cress, fennel, juniper, lettuce, mint, olive, onions, peony, rosemary, saffron, thyme, violets and willow.

Although botanists like joseph Banks and Carl von Linne (Linnaeus) are associated with botanical classification, the first efforts to organize plants systematically are attributed to the Greek, Theophrastus. He was born in 372 BC and became a close friend and scientific colleague of Aristotle. Among more than 200 books he wrote during his 82 years was the *Historia Plantarum* (History of Plants), which lists hundreds of medicinal plants and became a standard text for the next 1200 years. He was one of the first writers to dismiss the magic rituals associated with the harvest and preparation of herbal plants. He is known as the father of botany.

Greek medicine was famous throughout the Mediterranean and with the fall of the Greek and rise of the Roman Empire during the last two hundred years BC, the Romans began giving special citizenship to valued Greek physicians. Notable among these immigrants was Dioscorides. He was a Greek who lived in the first century AD. As a physician to emperors and armies he had plenty of opportunity to travel the plant kingdom.

He is said to have been private physician to Nero. His great work, *De Materia Medica,* contains 600 medicinal plants with details on the time of day for harvesting them at their most active, as well as how to grow, harvest and store herbs. This book dominated Roman medicine at the time and European herbal medicine for the next 1500years. Many of its recommendations have been verified today. He saw white willow *(Salix alba)* as a remedy for gout, used garlic against worms, and identified juniper berries correctly as a means of contraception. Other recognizable herbs he favoured included aloes, cabbage, roses, and senna pods.

Shortly after so great a herbalist as Dioscorides came Galen, another Greek, whose output and fame proved greater still. He lived from 129 AD until 199 and made a unique mark on medical knowledge. He followedthe Hippocratic idea ofthe four humours and classified all his medicines by their degree of influence on the humours. A heating herb of the third degree was hotter than one heating to only the first degree. He also embarked on what is now called polypharmacy - the inclusion of many different drugs in one medicine. A medicine could contain 50 to 100 different plants or minerals. Most of his writings were lost in a house fire, but his herbal knowledge survives as part of the work, *De Simplicibus.* This work was also a major influence on European medicine for the next 1300years until the upstart Paracelsus announced his own ascendancy with a public burning of Galen's book.

It is ironic that despite such a wealth of medical talent available to the Romans, public diseases like malaria were significant factors in the fall of the Roman Empire. The dark ages descended on Europe and Christianity dominated government and society. Science fell from grace and with it some of the precious historical records of medicine that could have altered our present understanding of the past, had they survived. In one destructive orgy, Christians sacked and burned the famous medical school at Alexandria with the total loss of the library of an estimated 700,000 books. This, of course, was before either mechanical printing or cheap paperbacks were invented, so there were no backup copies of most of these books.

During the dark ages monks, with their education and literary preoccupation, provided a refuge for herbal knowledge.

For nearly 600 years the monasteries were the main source of gathering and recording the use of plant medicines. Their knowledge of Latin and Greek, combined with their fondness for gardening, left them suitably qualified to translate the ancient Greek and Roman texts. The network of monasteries throughout Europe no doubt gave them good excuses and also the means to travel from one centre of learning to another, where they had the best access to texts and expert knowledge.

Monasteries have also been famed for the quality of their calligraphy and-book illustration, the copying of which they had turned into an art form as beautifully illustrated herbals. While the monks were in silent labour and Europe festered, the Arab nations were in the medical ascendancy again. The Arab, or Muslim empire was spreading through north Africa, collecting local medicinal knowledge and spreading Arab medicine which had been based largely on the ancient Greek schools. Twomajor figures emerged from the Arab world during the late dark ages. Rhazes was a noted physician in Baghdad who produced a large text which brought together medicinal knowledge from India, Greece, Syria and what was then Persia. Around 1,000 AD, Avicenna, who is the Hippocrates of the Arab world, produced his famous *Canon Medicinae*, which became a leading teaching text in medical schools for nearly 600 years. (His book was translated into Latin which was still the main language of learning, and which was in fact required for entry into Western medical schools until the 1960s.)

The late dark ages saw a flurry of herbals produced. The main reason for the outbreak was the repository of skills and interest within the monasteries. The first British herbal is the *Leech Book of Bald* written in the last years of the millennium. It combined foreign medical knowledge with local traditions. Later, in 1317, the *Rosa Anglica* was written by a monk drawing on ancient texts. Similar rewritings appeared across Europe.

As the Renaissance gave hope to a very depressed Europe, scientific thought and practice was encouraged once again. A Swiss with the improbable name of Philippus Aureolus Theophrastus Bombastus von Hohenheim reinvigorated herbal medicine in his peculiar and unique style. He was very arrogant and lived up to the 'bombast' part of his name. He is best known by his own choice of pen-name, Paracelsus meaning 'like Celsus', a much respected Roman physician. Paracelsus showed his dismissal of the ideas of Galen and Avicenna by publicly burning their books at the University where he lectured. He rejected the idea of multiple-ingredient medicines and the use of astrology, but revived the old Doctrine of Signatures and made it the focal point of his approach to medicine. He had great faith in nature's healing powers and is credited with the creation of laudanum, a preparation of opium, which was in popular medicinal use until the beginning of the twentieth century. Scientific herbals began to emerge like that of the English doctor, William Turner, in 1551. Gerard's *Herbal* appeared in 1597, William Cole's *The Art of Simpling* in 1656 and possibly the best-known of all herbals ever published, Culpeper's *Herbal,* in 1652. The Doctrine of Signatures was still influential and can be seen most clearly illustrated in Culpeper. He combined astrology with the Doctrine, but should be appreciated most for his radicalism in writing for the people. Until this time most medical books were kept in elitist Latin, partly to ensure that only the highly-educated physicians could access the treasures of information they contained. Culpeper's herbal was a deliberate act of defiance. He was training to be an apothecary, a profession that dispensed drugs but also acted as doctors to the poor who could not afford the physician's fees. Apothecaries served an apprenticeship rather than followed a University education, so they could not read the Latin texts. Culpeper translated the Latin tomes into English and wrote simply for ordinary people. His reward was the rage of the Royal College of Physicians who called him a 'most despicable ragged-fellow'.

The increasing popularity of herbal medicine during the sixteenth to eighteenth centuries had much to-do with the spread of apothecaries and the increasing popularity of accessible herbals and medical texts, especially with the invention of the printing press. The growing importation of herbs from foreign lands, especially from North America, also boosted interest as tales of their great merit spread in Europe.

The sixteenth century witnessed one of the most important events for modern herbalism in Britain: the so-called Quacks' Charter was passed in parliament. The events that led to this legislation are as relevant today as its impact on herbal medicine ever since. In the early decades the doctors were well-educated, privileged people with connections in high places. They also were well organized. One Thomas Linacre, personal doctor to King Henry VIII, set up the Royal College of Physicians and became its first president. Within a few years he had managed to get the King's blessings on a doctors' monopoly for treating the sick in and around London. This effectively banned herb women and other local healers from healing, even though the doctors were few in number and the poor could not afford their fees. There was also increasing rivalry between doctors and surgeons who were competing for patients, and between these groups and the barber surgeons whose services in minor operations are immortalized in the red and white barber's pole still seen today outside their shops. The apothecaries also created jealousy among the doctors, surgeons and barber surgeons. All these groups were fighting for the right to ask the public for money. A series of Acts of Parliament followed which divided up the diseases among the doctors' groups but extended their monopoly rights throughout the country. The more Acts were passed, the greedier the doctors and surgeons became, and the more pressure was put on the traditional herbalists to stop practicing. Of course, all this meant that the poor were losing their only source of healing. However, the greed seemed to eradicate political wisdom because one important herbalist's toes were trodden on too many times and he shouted loudly and effectively. This herbalist was Henry VIII.

Both Elizabeth I and her father Henry VIII were keen herbalists. Both had pride in their own inventions of formulae to cure their own ailments or those of fellow royals or courtiers around Europe. Perhaps Henry realized that the spreading monopoly of the doctors and surgeons also meant that he should not use herbs any more. The more likely motivation for his anger was his appreciation of traditional medicine and its importance for the common people. In 1543 he hit back with new legislation protecting the rights of common herbal healers.

The Act put the surgeons in their place with the accusation that they were more concerned 'with minding only their own lucre, and doing nothing for the profit or ease of the diseased or patient' and that in consequence they allowed the poor to 'rot and perish to death for lack of help'. The dramatic part of the Act was its overturning the efforts of the doctors to ban ordinary people from practicing herbal medicine. Henry's Act saw the rogue physicians and surgeons as persecutors of 'divers honest persons as well as men and women, whom God hath endowed with the knowledge of the nature, kind and operation of certain herbs, roots and waters'. Determined to correct affairs the Act decreed clearly that henceforth:

'it shall be lawful to every person being the King's subject, having the knowledge and experience of the nature of Herbs, Roots and Waters, or of the operation of the same, by speculation or practice within any part of the realm of England or within any other of the King's dominions, to practice, use and minister in an to any outward sore, uncome, wound, apostemations, outward swelling or disease, any herb or herbs, oyntments, baths, pultes and amplaisters, according to their cunning, experience and knowledge in any of the diseases sores and maladies beforesaid, and all other like to the same, or drinks for the Stone and Stanguary, or Agues, without suit, vexation, trouble, penalty, or loss of their goods.'

The Act was radical and still has influence. It recognized that a formal medical degree was not the only way to gain valuable knowledge about healing. In fact, such education was a form of de-education because it ignored both traditional local herbs and traditional understanding of illness and healing. The Act also listed all the main illnesses of the day and gave traditional healers the right to treat them as well as the doctors and surgeons. To this day, it is lawful in Britain for anyone to practice herbal medicine with relatively few restrictions. This right to use traditional herbs and healing skills has been outlawed in most other countries, where doctors have managed to ensure the suppression of traditional medicine, which King Henry VIII was farsighted enough to stop in the UK.

The nickname of Quacks' Charter was an attempt to put down the traditional healers by suggesting their skills and abilities were worthless and even harmful. It is interesting, that today herbal medicine has survived while many of the doctors' skills are being considered harmful and worthless. In the middle of the nineteenth century, leading herbalists like Coffin in North America and John Skelton in the English Midlands had established themselves as healing legends in their lifetime and the popularity of herbal medicine rocketed.

It was not until the twentieth century was 30 years old that herbal medicine began to fall into relative decline. Herbs were not discredited or shown to be ineffective. The reason was the coincidence of two well-matched phenomena. First, the squalor of industrial European cities encouraged the spread of infectious diseases which were the most common causes of illness and death. Second, the demand for medicines during the Second World War was frustrated by a shortage of natural medicines.

This gave great impetus to the development of new drugs by harnessing new skills in chemistry and pharmacy. The pharmaceutical industry took off and the impact of antibiotics such as penicillin and the sulphonamides made such a dramatic improvement in the chances of surviving infectious disease, that the herbal medicine was kicked into the role of a second-rank medicine.

My own father's experience is an interesting case. His father, his uncle, and his grandfather were all herbalists working in a clinic, The Botanic Institute, in Brisbane, Australia. He was set to follow in their footsteps in 1935. However, he was so struck with the stories of the new antibiotics that he felt the new medicine must be better than herbs. In 1938 he was accepted into the Faculty of Medicine at the University of Queensland, Brisbane. He practiced as a general practitioner for 40 years but became increasing skeptical of the wisdom of modern drugs and never rejected the efficacy and safety of herbs.

As recently as 1945, nearly three-quarters of all drugs used by doctors were herbal medicines. As the pharmaceutical industry expanded rapidly it began using marketing methods that offered doctors valuable inducements to use their drugs. Doctors took the carrots and turned to the 'modern' drugs while shunning herbal drugs. That the side effects of these modern drugs were often as severe as the symptoms doctors were treating was either ignored or seen as a justifiable cost of such effective medicine.

The marketing methods of drug companies have been regularly criticized. One study of British doctors' prescribing patterns showed a close relationship between the drugs being advertised in the *British Medical Journal* and the drugs prescribed by its readers. Such studies, plus the knowledge that doctors were treated by drug company representatives to 'friendly gestures' like expensive lunches, holidays abroad and even computers, has led to a clamp-down on such unacceptable practices.

Over the last two decades there has been growing concern with the path of Western medicine. Despite the jealously guarded superiority of the medical profession, it is increasingly clear that Western medicine is no panacea. Both diagnostic techniques and treatments are becoming more sophisticated, but there are few new breakthroughs or cures. The main causes of death in the West, heart disease and cancer, are still incurable and common debilitating diseases like rheumatoid arthritis, psoriasis and backache must be suffered stoically in the absence of cures or effective preventive measures. AIDS is the most fashionable incurable disease of the age and the lack of a cure is a real threat to the world's population.

The main criticism of orthodox medicine is not that it has failed to cure every human illness, but that it has insisted on following too narrow an approach despite ample evidence that its achievements are matched by its failures. Both public and, increasingly, doctors are now looking beyond the orthodox.

They are looking at alternative approaches to health and disease and to different ways of treating disease. There are many reasons for this. The failures to treat or cure illness, plus the high rate of side effects from orthodox treatments, worry doctors as much as patients.

But perhaps the patients are providing the strongest impetus for change. They are rejecting the way doctors treat them as people as much as they are rejecting the drug treatments. Most of the acceptable alternative approaches are already available in the community, and most are older than orthodox medicine.

Herbal medicine is becoming popular again. It should be seen not as an alternative system of medicine, but as one that is perfectly complementary. Our great legacy of traditional herbal knowledge is being constantly sifted, searched and interpreted for use in our time. The latest scientific research and other approaches to understanding health and disease are studied by herbalists and useful advances are incorporated into their pool of knowledge. The ancient and distinguishing hallmarks of herbal medicine are, however, retained: the use of plant medicines and the philosophy of finding and restoring the balance within the patient's whole body and .being.

Chapter Three

What Do Herbalists Treat?

There are popular misunderstandings about what you could present to a herbalist in reasonable expectation of successful treatment. The minimalists believe that only the simplest of conditions, like spots or indigestion, can be treated with herbs.

The great optimists feel that any illness at all should be presented to herbalists, especially if orthodox doctors have failed to treat it successfully. Both views are inadequate. What patients *do present* to herbalists for treatment is a different question, but one that helps clarify the subject of this chapter. Not all patients go first to a herbalist. Most patients see herbalists as a last resort after orthodox medicine, or even some other therapies, have failed. Herbalists see this as a challenge, not an insult. It means patients are bringing other practitioners' failures and it excites herbalists to take on these sometimes difficult cases and end up with happy, healed patients. But it does mean that herbalists are sometimes seen as useful *only* for difficult, chronic conditions like rheumatism, irritable bowel syndrome, adult acne, or the constant period pains and premenstrual symptoms that many women have been told are 'normal'. Herbalists are good with these chronic complaints, but that is not all. More and more patients are seeing their herbalist as their first point of call in both treating illness and staying healthy.

In practice, herbalists treat a very wide range of conditions.

Rather than produce a long list that would read like a medical dictionary, it is more useful to focus first on the factors that decide what a herbalist can treat. In short, there are three issues: the skill of herbalists in diagnosis, the range of healing actions available in medicinal plants, and the aim or purpose of treatment.

Herbalists who are members of the UK's National Institute of Medical Herbalists are trained very like doctors. They study the same anatomy, physiology and pathology. They also learn the same diagnostic tools and methods of physical examination.

While herbalists aren't doctors and will not pretend to be, they have the same basic skills. Herbalists are also trained to refer patients to GPs or other practitioners where necessary. This means you could take to a herbalist almost any condition you would take to a Doctor. British law states that only doctors are allowed to treat venereal disease and vets to diagnose or treat animals, but these exceptions leave wide scope for herbalists.

If herbalists diagnose certain serious conditions they will normally refer the patient to a GP or hospital. Anyone with symptoms of appendicitis, stroke or heart attack would be referred straight to hospital. Patients with serious acute conditions that may require hospitalization, special drug regimens, or specialist attention would normally be referred to their GP in the first instance. Patients with signs of serious diseases like kidney infection, diabetes or cancer, or of high blood pressure, would normally be encouraged to see their GP, even while they are seeing the herbalist. Many of these conditions are treatable with herbal remedies and herbalists often treat patients in conjunction with GPs or hospital consultants.

There is an extraordinary range of medicinal actions available from the 2,000 plants worldwide that are used as medicine. Most herbalists would use around 200 herbs in their own practice. Apart from the well-known actions of killing microbes, easing indigestion, and soothing itchy rashes, plants have useful effects like stimulating the body's hormones, increasing urine production, altering the heart's pumping action, increasing bile production or flow, relaxing muscle tension in internal organs, and calming an over-excited brain.

In fact, herbalists have access to medicinal plants for almost any condition they want to treat. Usually a single herb has more than one useful action and herbalists have a choice of combinations of actions. Chapter 5 discusses herbal medicines in more detail.

What is a treatment? Ideally it offers a cure, but it might also be aimed only at relieving symptoms in untreatable or chronic illness, or at preventing an illness from appearing or from recurring. The herbalist's approach tackles all stages of disease and is not limited to removing the immediate symptoms. With acute childhood eczema, for example, a herbalist might provide a cream which relieves the itching, treat internally to stop the cause of the rash, and offer preventive advice to help ensure that, once the cause is removed, the eczema does not return.

Some diseases like rheumatoid arthritis are very difficult to cure, but herbalists can do much to relieve the pain and swelling which make the condition so difficult to bear.

Sometimes a patient might require treatment from another therapy as well as herbal medicine. Recommendation of such treatments and their coordination with herbal treatment are both part of the benefits of seeing a herbalist. An example is someone with irritable bowel syndrome due to a history of family stress and job problems that caused anxiety or depression. The herbalist might treat the anxiety and irritable bowel with herbs but also' encourage the patient to see a counselor and have regular relaxing massages as well.

If in doubt, ask a herbalist. Most will offer a short, free consultation where you can outline your problems and the herbalist will say whether herbal treatment is likely to help.

These short consultations do not allow a full understanding or diagnosis, but give both the prospective patient and the herbalist a good idea of what to expect.

The following list shows some of the common conditions, affecting the main systems of the body, which herbalists treat.

Other conditions are treated, but they are either less common or are treated in close cooperation with the patient's GP.

System	Common Conditions Treated
Digestive	Mouth ulcers, gingivitis, bleeding gums, toothache, teething pains, oesophagitis, reflux oesophagitis, hiatus hernia, gastritis,' minor food poisoning, gastroenteritis, indigestion, peptic ulcer, liver and gall bladder disease, hepatitis, Crohn's disease, ulcerative colitis, constipation, diarrhoea, diverticulitis, irritable bowel syndrome (colitis), piles, anal fissure, worms, anal itching, obesity, nutritional deficiencies.
Respiratory	Colds, rhinitis, catarrh, hay fever, allergic rhinitis, sinusitis, bleeding nose, sore throat, irritable coughs, tonsillitis, quinsy, pharyngitis, laryngitis, bronchitis, asthma, bronchiecstasis, lung infections.
Circulatory	Chilblains, poor circulation in hands and feet, anaemia, raised blood pressure, angina, varicose veins, varicose eczema, piles, therosclerosis.
Urine and genital	Urinary tract infections of ureters and bladder, kidney stones, cystitis, bed wetting, enlarged prostate, minor infections of penis and vagina, vaginal discharges, thrush, painful periods, premenstrual syndrome, menopause.

Muscles and joints	Rheumatoid arthritis, osteoarthritis, fibrositis, myositis, housemaid's knee, tennis elbow, frozen shoulder, sprains, damaged ligaments and tendons.
Skin	Bites, stings, eczema, psoriasis, urticaria, drug and allergic eruptions, warts, whitlows, ingrown toenails and nail infections, herpes simplex and zoster (shingles), ringworm, acne, impetigo, thrush, tinea and other fungal infections, seborrhoea, dandruff, scabies, lichen planus, itchy anus and vagina, minor burns, sunburn.
Nervous	Simple anxiety, stress, insomnia, depression, functional digestive disturbances, migraine, tension headaches, recovery from stroke, post-viral syndrome, ME.
Ears, eyes	Excess wax, infections of outer ear canal, otitis media, glue ear, eustachian catarrh, tinnitus, conjunctivitis, conjunctival ulcer, blepharitis, styes.

Chapter Four

What Happens in a Consultation?

Many people would like to see a herbalist but delay making
the first appointment because they are uncertain of what to
expect in a consultation. While the rooms and equipment
will be familiar, the length and nature of the consultation are
different from most people's experience of doctors: these
differences are often the main reason why herbalists are
consulted.

Just to enter the clinic is reassuring because they look not
unlike any other clinic. There is usually a waiting room with a
friendly receptionist and even the familiar pile of out-of-date
magazines. Relaxing prints of interesting plants or luxuriant
green country scenery may hang on the walls.

Once welcomed into the consulting room, a quick glance
around is comforting, and will reveal nothing strange in the
layout or tools of the trade. There is likely to be a desk and
chair, an examination couch with a comforting blanket
folded at the foot, a pair of scales and a washbasin. The desk
may be decorated with the typical medical instruments you
see in any visit to your doctor - a sphygmomanometer for
measuring blood pressure, an ophthalmoscope and otoscope
for looking into the eyes and ears respectively, and a
stethoscope. In one corner or through an adjoining door you
can expect to see a dispensary where rows of bottles of
tinctures, jars of creams, and large containers of colourful
and odoriferous herbs are laid out in readiness for your
personal prescription to be dispensed.

By now your herbalist will have introduced him- or herself, shaken your hand and led you to your chair by the desk, which is where the differences begin. You will probably notice that you are not separated from the herbalist by the desk. You are most likely to be sitting on the same side of it, beside each other.

Holistic medicine is listening and talking medicine. It is essential that you and the practitioner feel as comfortable as possible with each other as soon as possible. The desk should be for writing on and displaying vases of flowers, and not used as a barrier.

The next difference is the length of a consultation. The first consultation takes from an hour to an hour and a half, so be prepared for this if you leave a car parked outside, for example!

Most of this time you will be talking and the herbalist will be listening, taking notes and asking questions to get the fullest picture of your concerns. Often this is the longest period the patient has ever spent talking about their health and it is normally enjoyed thoroughly. Follow-up appointments usually last half an hour.

The consultation itself is the most important part of your herbal treatment. Getting to the bottom of your health concerns means a more complete and more accurate diagnosis of the causes, 'which is essential for choosing the best treatment.

Herbalists will differ in how they approach a consultation, but all will tailor their routine to the immediate needs of each patient. A typical consultation would include detailed discussion on the following.

Content of a Typical Consultation with a Herbalist	
Presenting complaint	Patient describes in own words the symptoms or health concern that initiated the appointment. Questions on when first started, how long it has been there, what makes it better or worse; any treatments that have been tried and their level of success. Any other conditions that are present but may not be the main concern of the patient will also be asked about.
Previous medical history	A list of other diseases, accidents etc. will be sought, from childhood to the present. (Previous conditions may throw light on weakness, susceptibilities and even the presenting symptoms.)
Family history	Detailed check of the health of parents, brothers and sisters, and children of patient throws light of the presence of hereditary diseases or tendencies (e.g. rheumatoid arthritis, heart disease, allergies).
Previous drugs	You may be asked to recall pharmaceutical drugs taken within the previous two to ten years. This information can help identify earlier diagnoses, may explain some current symptoms from drug side-effects or reactions, and alerts the herbalist to any possible interactions with herbal medicines. 'Drugs' here also include aspirin, vitamin supplements, laxatives etc., which are bought without a prescription.

	Herbalists will often ask patients to prepare a list of these drugs before the first visit or bring the drug containers if that is easier. Our memory of drugs is usually poor and important omissions are too easy.
Lifestyle	Understanding of the patient's environment and their interaction with it is essential. Questions about smoking and drinking habits, type and frequency of exercise, hobbies and methods of relaxation are basic. Contentment in relationships, and with social life and work will be discussed.
Diet	Eating pattern and habits say much about health. A brief diet history will be taken, often starting with recall of everything eaten or drunk in the previous 24 hours. If diet is considered important to the immediate concerns, patients may be asked to keep a diet diary over 3-5 days after the first visit. Analysis may throw light of the condition or indicate specific changes that will improve health.
Body systems	Each of the body's main systems will be checked by simple questioning to check the underlying health of the whole body. The heart and circulation, respiratory system, digestion, nervous system, urinary and reproductive systems, skin, and muscles and joints will be checked one by one. Here the herbalist is looking for any

	indications that a system is not performing as it should be.
Reproductive system	Periods will be discussed to see they are regular and trouble free. Discharges, infections, pains, fertility, and difficulties with menopause will be raised as appropriate. Male fertility, infections and prostate problems will be checked.
Physical examination	So far only words have been exchanged. It is often valuable to examine affected parts of the body physically to get a clear picture of what is happening. Always with the patient's permission, examination might be of the circulation, lungs, abdomen, skin, muscles or joints as necessary. The findings are recorded in words and often simple drawings indicating any lumps, pain, sounds or tenderness.
Tests and measurement	Often simple tests are taken to help in the diagnosis or simply to record the state of the patient's health. These include urine tests, blowing into a tube (respirometer) to measure efficiency of breathing, measuring blood pressure, weighing. If blood tests are needed the patient is usually referred to their GP or sent to a laboratory where samples can be taken. If an X-ray, or similar test, is thought useful the patient may be referred to their GP.

At the end of the history part of the consultation, the herbalist usually has reached one of more conclusions about the diagnosis. This involves not only identifying the medical nature of the problem the patient came with, but what caused it. These findings are usually discussed at length with the patient so that the nature and total causes of the condition are fully understood.

Herbalists are not content to give only a diagnosis. As part of their approach to healing, they usually devote plenty of time to explaining and discussing any diagnosis with their patient. How can the patient be expected to work at restoring the function and balance within their body without having some understanding of what has gone wrong and of the herbalist's strategy for restoring it to health? Knowledge is power and power is healing.

Sometimes it may not be possible to reach a clear diagnosis at the first visit, or there may be several possibilities. This is normal. There are common conditions, like inflammatory bowel disease or rheumatoid arthritis, where experts dispute the diagnosis even after a battery of tests and investigations. And of course there are conditions like ME (myalgic encephalomyelitis) whose very existence is disputed as much as the criteria for its diagnosis. It is good medical practice to keep the possibilities of a firm diagnosis open until all the reasonable alternatives have been eliminated. Herbal treatment is well adapted to such an open mind because not only are patients monitored carefully during treatment, but herbalists normally modify their medication regularly as the patient progresses. In this way, alternative diagnoses can be borne in mind and eliminated as more information is shared by patient and practitioner.

Once the diagnosis has been discussed, the proposed treatment is presented. I say 'presented' because herbalists recognize that the patient must agree with the treatment if it is to be followed. It is usual for a herbalist to propose several elements of treatment apart from the obvious herbal medicine.

For example, there may be dietary change, increased levels of exercise, encouragement for a change of job, or a holiday for two on a tropical island without the children *plus* a course of herbal medicine. All of these may be desirable for better health but the patient may find some proposals either impractical or simply unlikely to be followed. Few patients can take off on the much-needed holiday the day after their consultation, but many more just don't want to take up simpler measures like following a healthier diet. Herbalist and patient enter into negotiation.

Both are aiming to agree on the successful blend of what the herbalist considers will restore and maintain health with what the patient feels they can stick to. This is a process, not a dispute.

Because the herbalist is tailoring any treatment to the individual patient's needs through discussion, what is proposed and what is accepted are usually remarkably close. Herbal medicines may be part of treatment. At the end of the consultation, a prescription is designed specifically for that patient. Whether a cream, tincture or tea, this prescription may contain anything from one to ten or more herbal ingredients.

A single prescription may be designed to affect several organs or systems of the body according to the strategy for healing.

Herbalists dispense their own medicines on site. An important feature of herbal medicines is that the herbalist will review and modify prescriptions at each visit. This allows the medication to be modified as needed to follow the improving patient's changing needs.

Follow-up visits are usually for 30 minutes. Frequency and the total number of visits required vary with the condition. Most herbalists arrange their first follow-up for two weeks after the first visit. This is soon enough to see any initial effects of treatment and allows for other information like diet diaries, blood tests etc. to be available to help refine the diagnosis and hence treatment. Subsequent visits may be monthly. Although it is difficult to generalize about how many visits will be needed, between 4 and 8 visits is a good working average. Some conditions may require only one, whereas long-standing chronic conditions may take more.

Chapter Five

What Are Herbal Medicines?

Pharmacists and doctors tend to see a medicine as
something produced in a modern and sophisticated factory,
available in purified form, and provided in precisely
measured doses. They see herbal medicines as not only
different from but not even compatible with their modern
medicines; as medicines that are neither dispensed by
pharmacists nor prescribed by doctors.

Herbalists or members of the public tend to see herbal
medicines as the use of whole plant material or simple
extracts.

They also see their 'herbs' as distinctly different from
pharmaceutical drugs; many people prefer them to the
exclusion of modern drugs. Both views offer only an
incomplete description, one which does not help our
understanding of these medicinal gifts from nature.

The term 'herbal medicine' can be applied to a broad
spectrum of medicines. There is no generally accepted
definition, partly because different professional interests
choose not to agree. However, there are clear facts about the
use of plants as medicine that help us reach a versatile and
helpful basic definition.

One reason to conserve the tropical rainforests is the work
done by the large numbers of scientists who are known as
ethnobotanists. They are scurrying around on the forest
floor looking for new sources of drugs, not as plants for
high-street herbalists but as raw materials for the
pharmaceutical industry.

Of the 40 per cent of all modern drugs that are derived from plants, some are isolated extracts of plant material and others are synthetic copies of active ingredients found in plants. Many of our most valuable modern drugs come from plants. Antibiotics are derived from fungi, which are plants. Heart drugs like digoxin, the most-used heart stimulant drug, and reserpine come from plants. *Cantharanthus roseus* (Madagascar periwinkle) provided one of the first effective treatments for childhood leukaemias. Strong sedatives and painkillers like morphine come from poppies. Liquorice extract is used to treat peptic ulcers, while senna pods, ispaghula husks, cascara, phenol, and witch hazel are all used in modern drugs for various bowel problems. It hardly seems appropriate for the pharmaceutical industry or doctors to hide their reliance on plant medicines.

Herbalists, however, are more easily identified with the use of plant medicines. It is in their name and in their blood. They often describe their medicines simplistically as 'whole plants'.

This is not strictly true. Unless a plant is consumed root, branch and tops, it isn't the 'whole plant' that is being used. Usually it is the specific parts of a medicinal plant that are used for their particular concentration of active ingredients - the green shoots or flowers of herbaceous plants, or flowers, or bark, or roots.

The most used forms of herbal medicine are teas (infusions) and tinctures. Both are crude extracts which contain the desired active ingredients. Herbal teas are made just like ordinary Indian or Chinese tea, but are drawn or infused for 10-15 minutes instead of only 3-5 minutes. Once the soluble extract is released from the plant material, the tea is strained and the solid residue is *thrown away*, not consumed. Tinctures are made in a similar process where solutions of alcohol (or glycerol) and water are used to extract ingredients that are less soluble in water alone. Again the residue is thrown away. The whole plant is rarely used. (There are exceptions, such as taking herbs in powdered form in gelatine capsules. These and other forms of herbal medicine are discussed below under 'preparations'.)

Thus both herbalists and the modern pharmaceutical drugs use extracts of plant materials. It makes sense therefore to include in our basic definition of herbal medicines; *medicine that uses plant material, crude extracts of plants or isolates of ingredients from plants.* That includes the wide scope of plant use in medicines but there are very important differences in the type of extract taken and in how the medicine is formulated. These differences make clear the distinction between herbal medicine from a herbalist and herbal medicine from the pharmaceutical industry.

Herbal Extracts

The herbalist extracts all the soluble material from a plant. Plants contain thousands of different chemicals and, depending on their solubility, a large proportion of them are contained in the crude extract and hence in the herbal medicine. Medicinal plants are chosen for their relatively high concentration of the particular chemicals that are the healing agents. Only rarely is a single chemical thought responsible for the healing action.

Plants that have only one notable action usually contain a series of responsible chemicals. Gentian *(GentiaM lutea)* is used only for its renowned bitter action (see page 69), but this is due to the presence of several groups of chemicals - like iridoids and alkaloids. Oak bark is one of the best astringent remedies for use on the skin. This property is due to the high tannin content, > but tannins are a complex mixture of substances, not a single chemical.

Many plants contain a range of substances, which give related or supporting actions, thus making the whole remedy more complete and effective. For example, marshmallow *(Althaea officinalis)* and comfrey *(Symphytum officinale)* roots are valuable protective, soothing and healing remedies, being particularly rich in mucilages. The mucilages are special forms of carbohydrate that readily dissolve in water to produce a slimy texture. However, it is rare for the medicinal value of a plant to rest on only one chemical. These two plants both contain other chemicals that contribute to their healing actions. Comfrey, for example, also contains the anti-inflammatory rosmarinic acid and alantoin, which- hastens the healing of wounds and even broken bones.

A more striking example of the range of actions and contributing chemicals in one plant is seen with the popular herbal tea, chamomile *(Matricaria retutita)*. In general use, this is drunk as a digestive or calming hot drink. Many drink it for its taste alone. But herbalists recognize it as an antispasmodic to relax the intestines, as a digestive in flatulence and indigestion, as a mild sedative, as an anticatarrhal, as an anti-inflammatory in eczema, leg ulcers and haemorrhoids, and as an excellent remedy to reduce nausea in travel sickness and morning sickness. These actions come from a mixture of chemicals including volatile oils (the strong smell and taste of chamomile tea), flavonoids, bitter glycosides, and tannins. Even among the volatile oils are different component oils that are responsible for the relaxing and anti-inflammatory actions.

Often the renowned success of a herbal medicine depends on the interaction of its chemicals or the combined effects of several active ingredients. Sometimes the active chemicals have never been identified, even though the medicinal properties of a plant have been known for years. For example, vitamin C or ascorbic acid is recognized as one of our essential vitamins. It is found naturally in many plants including fruits, berries and many green leaves. In the past, sailors took lemons and limes to sea to prevent scurvy. Little did they know that it wasn't only the vitamin C in the lemons that protected them but also a companion chemical, the bioflavonoids. Although isolated, purified vitamin C is sold as a vitamin supplement and given to mothers for their babies, much research has shown that vitamin C is most effective when used in the natural combination with bioflavonoids. Some studies even showed that scurvy, one disease caused by deficiency of the vitamin, was not cured with vitamin C alone, but only when lemon extract was given. To call the English 'limeys' is to mock them. Perhaps the term should be used as a mark of respect for their unconscious wisdom.

Much is known about how herbal medicine works, but that covers only a fraction of the outstanding questions. It is easier to study the behavior of drugs based on single chemicals like modern pharmaceutical drugs. Herbal medicines are more difficult because they are much more complex mixtures. In most cases, only a fraction of the plant's chemical constituents have been identified. This makes it difficult to predict how a plant drug may work. However, there have been many studies on how these complex combinations of chemicals affect health. Time and again it has been shown that plants have healing actions far greater than might be predicted from the known concentration of active ingredients. The whole action is greater than the sum of the component parts.

Pharmaceutical Drugs and Herbal Medicines

A pharmaceutical drug differs from a herbal extract in three main aspects. First, it is made of a single chemical substance which may be of plant, mineral or animal origin. Single chemical substances may be isolated from plant extracts, be synthetic copies or be slightly altered copies. There may also be bulking agents, a sugar coating or some other substance which merely helps the active chemical get into the body. Second, the extract is purified and available as a medicine in much higher doses than could be achieved with most herbal medicines.

Third, the doses are metered precisely so the doctor knows the precise amount of medicine the patient gets.

Isolated extracts behave very differently from the whole plant extract, and not always to the benefit of the patient. The foxglove *(Digitolis purpurea)* contains several cardioactive glycosides, which are active against the heart muscle. Their effect is to help a failing or aged heart pump more efficiently. Isolated single glycosides like digoxin are widely-used heart drugs. They are very useful, but also cause many poisonings, because the effective dose is very close to the toxic dose and digoxin is lost from the blood only slowly. However, in the natural plant extract, the glycosides are associated with other chemicals that control their availability and thus make poisoning less likely.

Because of this interaction, only a tenth of the digoxin in the form of the plant extract is needed to produce the same effect on the heart as the purified glycoside used alone in a pharmaceutical drug. The risk of poisoning is greatly reduced while the patient has the same benefit to the heart.

Lily-of-the-valley. *(COfWallaria majalis)* is another plant herbalists value for heart disease. It too contains cardioactive glycosides, the most important of which are called convallatoxin and convallatoxol. Again, the natural mixture of plant constituents is superior to the isolated chemicals. The former is rapidly active, increasing the strength of the heart action.

The second is conveniently converted into the more active convallatoxin as it is used up in the heart muscle. This means that the effective action of the herb is prolonged without increasing the dose. Other chemicals in the whole plant extract act to increase the solubility, and hence availability in the body, of the heart-affecting chemicals by a factor of 500. Again this means that less of the active chemical is needed for a beneficial effect and the risk of poisoning is greatly reduced.

There is often merit in purifying active ingredients, but there is no sense in insisting that only isolates should be used as medicines. Aspirin is a good example. The anti-inflammatory and pain-relieving properties of the salicylates were discovered from studies of meadowsweet and white willow *(Salix alba)*. The modern drug is a synthetic version of the natural chemical.

Aspirin is *acetyl* salicylate which is a slightly modified version of a natural chemical. They behave differently in the body. Aspirin is more concentrated, but it has an unfortunate tendency to irritate the lining of the stomach wall so much that bleeding is often caused. Fatal bleeding caused by aspirin is not unknown. The natural form does not irritate the stomach at all, and indeed is used to treat irritations of the stomach and intestine.

Precise doses are a misleading benefit of pharmaceutical drugs. Of course, with toxic drugs it is useful to know how much is being given in a dose. But that does not mean there can be no toxic effects. Many doctors are reluctant to prescribe digitoxin because toxic effects are so common on the recommended doses.

It is wrong to believe that a precise dose is the same thing as the exact dose needed for a particular patient. The dosages recommended to doctors are based on trials with different patients and are a rough average figure. By definition of the average, many patients will need higher amounts to get the benefits. For many people the average dose will be too much and they may suffer unnecessary side effects because the recommended dose is close to toxic for them. A precise dose often means little in reality. Antidepressive drugs are an example where the effect on a patient is so unpredictable that doctors often spend weeks or months adjusting. dosage up and down while also trying different drugs in the hope of achieving the desired effect.

It is much more difficult to be precise about the concentration of any ingredient in a plant medicine. Plants are natural materials. Their composition varies with many factors including soil type and climate, time of harvest, conditions of storage and method of preparation of the medicine. However, the dose of a herbal medicine is normally less critical than with pharmaceutical drugs. The herbalist's skill is knowing how much of each herb to give for the desired response. Usually the response is quickly detected because herbalists work by beginning with in-depth case histories, they see patients regularly to monitor progress, and they modify, or fine tune, their medicines to keep up with the patient's needs. Overdosing is less of a problem because, with few exceptions, herbal remedies are very dilute and also have a low toxicity,

But herbal medicines are chosen to do work differently in the body from pharmaceutical drugs. The actions of herbs tend to be more supportive of normal healthy bodily functions and processes, whereas other drugs tend to be more suppressive of normal functions so any excess dose is expected to be more of a problem.

In one sense herbs are more like foods than drugs. Foods are eaten for the nutrients and other substances they contain, all of which support normal growth, functioning, muscle movement, repair 'of tissues, and reproduction. Although there is a minimum amount of each nutrient needed for healthy bodies, no one eats a diet that contains precisely the required amount, or dose, of each nutrient. Nor is this only because such a diet would be very boring. It is because, within wide limits, the body takes what it needs from the diet and harmlessly disposes of the excess. Who worries about eating a precise amount of vitamin C or protein? No one. Even when taking a vitamin supplement, the precise dose is rarely of consequence. (Exceptions to this simple comparison are the tendency to get fat if too many calories are eaten, and poisoning if very large amounts of fat-soluble vitamins A and D are eaten over many months.)

Herbal medicines range across a wide spectrum. At one extreme, dosage matters little, and at the other it is critical.

Many herbal medicines are also foods (garlic, pineapple, apricot, artichoke, ginger, liquorice) and dosage has little precision. Towards the middle are herbs like the laxatives (senna, yellow dock), mucous membrane tonics (plantain, golden seal, ground ivy) or the relaxing nervines (valerian, hops, Californian poppy), where the dose must be carefully chosen to achieve the desired effect. Too much or too little can be unsatisfactory. At the extreme end are herbs which are very potent: indeed, many are covered by the Poisons Act and even herbalists must pay scrupulous attention to dosage. Herbs like belladonna *(Atropa belladfmna)*, monkshood *(Aconitum napellus)*, and henbane *(Hyoscyamus niger)* are typical examples. Another herb in this critical dosage group is chilli *(Capsicum minimum)*, which is not a poison but is so hot that adding any more than the smallest measured dose will render the medicine totally unpalatable.

Herbs as Medicine

Here it is important to be sure some basic concepts are clear and understood, or a full appreciation of herbal medicines will never be reached. All of us in industrial countries have been brought up in a world of pharmaceutical drugs. These are usually single-ingredient drugs with one target action in the body. There are, of course, other effects, which are usually unplanned and are undesirable - they are called side effects. Steroid drugs, for example, are normally used to suppress inflammation in the body but their unwanted side effects include diabetes, osteoporosis, raised blood pressure, thinning
of the skin, unwanted hair growth, and depression. Herbal medicines are totally different. They have many ingredients and each herb usually has several or many different actions in the body. These multiple actions are of fundamental importance to how herbs work and how they are used by a herbalist. Herbs may also have side effects, but these are normally so minor that they are unnoticed (see chapter 6).

Some people find these important differences hard to grasp, or at least to adopt. An example will help illustrate the problems.

Recently I was discussing natural medicines with publishers who were interested in another book on the relationship between natural medicines like herbs and pharmaceutical drugs made from natural medicines. They were so used to the one substance - one action character of pharmaceutical drugs that they thought I was mistaken and confused when I showed them some text listing both multiple ingredients and actions for single herbs. They tried to cross out all but one ingredient and one action! After long explanation they reluctantly accepted my text represented the facts, but I suspect never really understood the concept. This was confirmed later when they insisted on describing herbs as *ingredients* of pharmaceutical drugs. They seemed to have great difficulty understanding not only that modern drugs are only a single chemical, but that since they are often extracted from plants, the modern drugs should be described as ingredients of plants. To fail to grasp the differences is to fail to understand the essence of natural medicines.

Herbalists treat people, not symptoms. This means that herbs are chosen for their actions on the body rather than to treat a particular symptom. Of course, herbs can be used to relieve symptoms, but usually in the context of treating the whole body.

Herbs are chosen for a prescription on the basis of the total character of each herb. The mixture and the balance of the actions in a herb, as well as knowledge of the general temperament of the each herb, are the important considerations.

However, in order to understand how herbs work, we can consider some of the important constituents that contribute to the main actions.

Active Ingredients

There is a great diversity of types of chemicals in plants, and the list of identified individual chemicals runs to thousands. It is not only the more biologically active, like alkaloids, that are medicinally useful. Many relatively inactive substances, like the mucilages or tannins, are so useful that they have been extracted for use in pharmaceutical drugs. Bearing in mind the fact that herbalists use whole plant extracts, some of the more valuable types of constituents are described below.

PLANT ACIDS

Just thinking about sinking the teeth into the flesh of a juicy
lemon brings to mind such a clear picture of the fruit's
acidity that saliva flows freely in response. Several other
plants are strongly acid to the taste (sorrel, green apples,
rhubarb and citrus fruits). But all plants are rich in a variety
of simple acids, which are probably the most common
chemical type in plants.

Their acid taste is normally not apparent because the acids
are bound to other chemicals, which alters the taste.

The simplest acids include formic and acetic acid. Stinging
nettles rely on small hairs containing formic acid to produce
their familiar sting and rash. Acetic acid is produced when
the alcohol in wine is exposed to the air, making vinegar.
Oxalic acid is found in leaves of spinach, dock and rhubarb
and has a tendency to encourage the formation of kidney
stones if eaten in excessive amounts. Succinic and fumaric
acids are common in plants and have a laxative action
because they irritate the wall of the bowel. -

More complex acids include the fruit acids: tartaric, citric and
malic acids. These give fruits their sour taste and are gentle
but efficient laxatives, which explains in part why eating
plenty of fruit improves bowel function.

All plant cells contain vegetable oils. The cooking and salad oils to be found in every kitchen are known as fixed oils as distinct from the volatile oils discussed below. The fixed oils come from particularly rich parts of certain plants like peanuts, sunflower seeds and olive fruits. But every green leaf also contains oils in small quantities. All these oils contain acids called fatty acids. Some of these are so important for our health they are called 'essential fatty acids'. These are instantly recognized under the name polyunsaturated fatty acids and include linoleic and linolenic acids. There are also relatives called saturated fatty acids like myristic, stearic and palmitic acids, which are less beneficial to health and contribute to causing heart disease. All these fatty acids are found combined with other chemicals in plant oils which are useful for moisturizing and protecting the skin, as laxatives or purgatives (castor oil, for example), and for softening and removing ear wax. The Egyptians had a more-drastic use for cedar oil, which was pumped into bodies being prepared for mummification to dissolve away all the internal organs, leaving only a shell of skin and bones.

CARBOHYDRATES

Carbohydrates are most readily associated with excess calories and being overweight. Herbalists are fonder of them. All plants contain many different carbohydrates; in fact plants could be described as carbohydrate factories. There are the simple sugars like the fruit sugar, fructose, and glucose, which are among the first products of the photosynthesis reaction in green plants; the starches, which are the plant's way of storing energy; and the hemicelluloses and cellulose, which make up the cell walls that allow plants from dandelion flowers to giant redwood trees to stand erect.

The simple carbohydrates are soluble in water and easily digested in the gut to supply energy (calories). The longer chain carbohydrates are known as polysaccharides and are generally insoluble and indigestible. They have a variety of uses to herbalists. The same pectin used to set jams is water absorbent and indigestible, making it a useful bulking agent to ease the constipated bowel. Similar substances in the outer seed husks of flea seed form a soft gel when cold water is poured on to the seeds. The gel also helps keep a soft stool in the gut and improves bowel function. Fybogel and Isogel are made of flea seed husks.

Mucilage is of particular importance to -herbalists. This complex carbohydrate is slimy to feel. Its composition varies among plants, but it is the sliminess rather than the specific chemical constituents that is important. Mucilages coat mucous membranes with a protective coating. They are only partially digested so can travel throughout the intestines, providing protection to any irritated or inflamed tissues that they pass over. Not only does this coating relieve irritations like gastritis or colitis, it can also calm the intestines by protecting the sensitive nerve endings in the wall of the gut from contact with allergens in foods.

Mucilages also benefit the lungs and urinary tract, despite the fact that mucilage is not absorbed in the intestines. It works by reflex action. The lungs and urinary tract are closely related to the intestines in their origin in the growing embryo. This closeness has left connections in the nervous system between these organs so that stimulating the lining of the gut can produce effects in the lungs or urinary tract. When mucilage soothes the gut, the same relief is experienced in irritated lungs or the ureters by reflex. Thus dry irritated lungs, asthmatic spasm, the painful spasms or colic due to urinary gravel and stones, or even cystitis can be relieved.

PHENOLS

This potent group are special forms of alcohol based on the six carbon ring structure of benzene. The group contains some of the most widely available and most useful ingredients of medicinal herbs. Some are simple structures based on one or two rings joined together, but others are very complex.

The simple phenols include salicylic acid, which is the basis of aspirin. Close chemical relatives are found in plants like willow *(Salix alba)*, meadowsweet and poplars. It occurs as gaultherin (oil of wintergreen), which is an ingredient of many warming skin creams and liniments. Salicylates reduce fever, are strongly antiseptic, stimulate bile production in the liver and reduce pain and inflammation.

Many simple phenols are strongly antibacterial and antiworm. Phenol itself is one of the standards against which antiseptics are compared. On the skin the phenols are anaesthetic, caustic and vesicant, which means they cause blisters. Eugenol (clove oil) is anaesthetic (toothache), antifungal, antiseptic and antiworm as well as being heating to the skin, which 'makes it useful in treating inflammations like rheumatism or muscle strains. Thymol, which is found in thyme and its relatives, has similar properties.

More complex phenols include the valuable tannins. These are found throughout the plant world and most plants contain small amounts of some form of tannin. They are most recognizable in the barks and leaves of woodland trees like oaks, beech and witch hazel, but are found also in seeds, fruits and in the leaves of shrubs and small herbaceous plants. Many household foods contain appreciable amounts of tannins.

They have a characteristic effect of precipitating proteins, even when small amounts of tannin are present. This changes the molecules from soft flexible threads to a contracted, tough into. Tannins are soluble in water and the water-alcohol solutions most herbal tinctures are made from. Tannins are used to tan leather. The protein in the leather is turned into a tough mass which not only resists attack from insects and fungi, but also from the wear and tear of human usage. In healing internally, the precipitated proteins form a tough protective layer over inflamed or damaged membranes.

Tannins are used externally on burns and open wounds where they form a protective cover or 'eschar' holding the wound closed, keeping infective organisms at bay, and encouraging the natural healing processes to work. They can stop certain forms of diarrhoea by protecting the gut wall from irritants and, because of their effect on protein, are an effective antimicrobial.

Many poisonous alkaloids are also precipitated by tannins, which makes them a useful antidote to alkaloid poisoning. Coumarins are small but useful group of phenols. They are responsible for the alluring smell of new-mown hay or grass.

Grasses and the pea family of plants contain the most valuable sources. The group seems to have special affinity for the blood and the blood vessels themselves. Many coumarins are anticlotting agents and several have been isolated for use in pharmaceutical drugs. Close chemical relatives useful to herbalists include aesculetin in the horse chestnut and ash, and herniarin in lavender and rue. The group contains the strong blood vessel dilators, khellin and visnagin, from khella, *Ammi visnaga*. Sun lovers who cheat nature by opting for lotions containing the artificial-tanning aid, bergapten, can have the solace of knowing that the bergapten itself is natural. It is a coumarin derived from bergamot oil, the flavouring used in Earl Grey tea.

The anthraquinone derivatives of phenol supply some of the most effective stimulant laxatives and purgatives. (See actions below for discussion of other forms of laxatives.) They act by stimulating the natural, rhythmical muscle contractions in the gut wall, also known as peristalsis. They act 8-12 hours after taking the medicine and there is usually some uncomfortable tangle. This is what happens when hides are tanned to make leather. In the mouth this causes that dry, rough feel to the inner cheeks when strong black tea is drunk or, more dramatically, when an unripe persimmon or a piece of banana peel is bitten into. Tannins are soluble in water and the water-alcohol solutions most herbal tinctures are made from.

Tannins are used to tan leather. The protein in the leather is turned into a tough mass which not only resists attack from insects and fungi, but also from the wear and tear of human usage. In healing internally, the precipitated proteins form a tough protective layer over inflamed or damaged membranes.

Tannins are used externally on burns and open wounds where they form a protective cover or 'eschar' holding the wound closed, keeping infective organisms at bay, and encouraging the natural healing processes to work. They can stop certain forms of diarrhoea by protecting the gut wall from irritants and, because of their effect on protein, are an effective antimicrobial.

Many poisonous alkaloids are also precipitated by tannins, which makes them a useful antidote to alkaloid poisoning. Coumarins are small but useful group of phenols. They are responsible for the alluring smell of new-mown hay or grass. Grasses and the pea family of plants contain the most valuable sources. The group seems to have special affinity for the blood and the blood vessels themselves. Many coumarins are anticlotting agents and several have been isolated for use in pharmaceutical drugs. Close chemical relatives useful to herbalists include aesculetin in the horse chestnut and ash, and herniarin in lavender and rue. The group contains the strong blood vessel dilators, khellin and visnagin, from khella, *Ammi visnaga*. Sun lovers who cheat nature by opting for lotions containing the artificial-tanning aid, bergapten, can have the solace of knowing that the bergapten itself is natural. It is a coumarin derived from bergamot oil, the flavouring used in Earl Grey tea.

The anthraquinone derivatives of phenol supply some of the most effective stimulant laxatives and purgatives. (See actions below for discussion of other forms of laxatives.) They act by stimulating the natural, rhythmical muscle contractions in the gut wall, also known as peristalsis. They act 8-12 hours after taking the medicine and there is usually some uncomfortable griping associated with the stimulation so a herbal carminative is usually given at the same time. Key members of the group include rhein from the dock and cassia families of plants and aloe-emodin from the rhubarb and cassia families.

Senna pods, from the cassia family, provide the sennosides. These are very effective laxatives and are also used in many pharmaceutical laxative preparations.

The flavones and flavonoids are the most common phenols.

They are yellow,bitter substances often found in flowers, where they have a role in attracting pollinating insects. For the herbalist, they offer a range of useful actions. They are diuretic, muscle-relaxing, anti-inflammatory, and antiseptic. The group contains chemicals like apigenin in celery; quercitol, from which rutin is formed; kaempferol from elder and horsetail; and rotenone, from the roots of *Den-is elliptica,* which is a natural insecticide approved for use on organic crops. The bioflavonoids, also known as vitamin P, include rutin and hesperedin, which are particularly active in protecting the strength of blood vessel walls.

The flavanolignans are a mixture of flavones with lignan, the strong 'cement' that sticks plant cells together. They include a particularly useful chemical, silimarin, from the milk thistle *(Cardus marianus)* .. This protects liver cells from damage from toxins and seems to speed up the rate of repair of liver cells after diseases like hepatitis.

VOLATILE OILS

The smells from plants come from volatile oils. The seductive perfume of roses and the saliva-inducing aroma of chopped basil are both due to volatile oils. These are not single oils but complex mixtures of many chemicals, not all of which have been identified. They are as potent and varied in their medicinal uses to herbalists as they are varied in aroma and origin.

Chemically they are based on multiples of a chemical called a terpene which is made up of two molecules of a chemical with five carbon atoms. Different volatile oils have multiples of the five carbon units as 'building blocks'. The monoterpenes are the most widespread family, containing the most volatile oils. They are thus the most strongly aromatic and include oils like pinene, camphor, menthol, limonene and thujone. They are antiseptic, antifungal, antiworm, heating to the skin (rubifacient), expectorant, carminative and even diuretic. One member of the family, citronellal, is an insect repellent.

The next step upwards in complexity of volatile oils is the sesquiterpenes which includes an important group of antiinflammatory, antispasmodic and generally calming compounds including the azulenes from chamomile and yarrow (Achillea millefolium), and both disabolol and farnesene from chamomile. Over 60 sesquiterpenes have been shown to have antitumour activity, notably those found in the daisy family of plants, including arnica and some thistles. Many sesquiterpenes are also bitter, a property of great importance to herbalists (see under actions below). Among the terpenes in the complex mixture that makes up the volatile oils are a pot-pourri of related chemicals, which often have medicinal actions along with the terpenes. The sulphur-based smell of the mustard oils in cabbage and radish or the unique smell of garlic are obvious examples, both of which are greatly treasured by herbalists.

SAPONINS

As the group name might suggest, the saponins are .named after soap. They do tend to form a lather in water, but their other properties are more exciting. They are related to the terpenes in their chemical origins but have different and important properties. Two types are found. The steroidal saponins have a structure very similar to natural steroid hormones in animals.

As herbal drugs, many of them seem to mimic hormones in their action and thus produce valuable effects, especially on the female reproductive system. The closely related triterpenoid saponins are more useful to herbalists. They include the saponins in liquorice, Asiatic (Panax ginseng) and Siberian (Elutherococcus senticosus) ginsengs, horse chestnut and the sweet violet (Viola odorata). They have many useful actions including being anti-inflammatory, diuretic, sedative and expectorant.

They also mimic or stimulate human hormones. Most notable is their stimulation of the body's private internal supply of steroids, the glucocorticoids, which are produced by the body's adrenal glands. .

CARDIOACTIVE GLYCOSIDES

These have a specific action on the heart muscle and tend to increase both the strength and speed of the pumping action, thus helping a failing or weakened heart. The classic examples are digoxin and digitoxin from the foxglove *(Digitalis purpurea* and *D. Iantana)*. The most valuable heart herb in modern herbalists' dispensaries is the lily-of-the-valley *(Convallaria majalis)*, which is less toxic than the foxglove and has a more prolonged action.

Other plants containing these glycosides are the figwort *(Scrophularia rwdosa)*, squill *(Urginea maritima)*, and pheasant's eye *(Adonis vernalis)*.

CYANOGENIC GLYCOSIDES

In large amounts, these ingredients are toxic as they produce prussic acid. However, in the amounts usually contained in herbal medicines, they are both safe and valuable. They are sedative and relaxing to muscles. Amygdalin and prunasin from species of *Prunus* are used in cough suppressants, as they relax the irritating and useless cough reflex in dry, throaty coughs. The elder *(Sambucus nigra)* contains sambunigrin.

GLUCOSINOLATES

The brassicas, which include cabbage, horseradish and mustard, are rich in sulphur and nitrogenous compounds that supply the characteristic odours and hot taste of these plants.

Sinalbin and sinigrin are two of the most useful examples from mustard, rape and shepherd's purse *(Capsella bursa-pastoris)*. They are used on the skin as counter-irritants in inflammatory conditions. Internally they are antimicrobial and, in small doses, are digestive stimulants.

BITTER PRINCIPLES

A 'bitter' is just that, bitter to the taste. This seemingly simple characteristic is one on the most used and valuable actions of herbal medicines. The bitterness is sometimes unpleasant, but it has to be. Any attempt to disguise the taste cancels out the action. The bitter taste stimulates bitter receptors on the tongue and triggers a chain of reactions in the digestive tract. The treasured actions include stimulating the flow of saliva, the appetite, the release of digestive acids in the stomach, the production of bile in the liver and its release into the intestines, secretion of hormones by the pancreas, and the production of protective mucus in the stomach so the chances of developing ulcers are reduced, as well as increasing the tone of the openings from the stomach so leakage of contents up into the oesophagus is less likely. Many different substances supply bitterness and most herbs used as bitters have other actions, which are usually complementary in the total treatment strategy being followed by the herbalist. The monoterpenes and sesquiterpenes supply several particularly bitter substances such as gentiopicrin from gentian and centaury. Many alkaloids are also bitter and are found in notable bitter remedies like barberry *(Berberis vulgaris)*, golden seal *(Hydrastis canadensis)* and quinine *(Cinchona succirubra)*.

ALKALOIDS

Although these represent only a part of the medicinally useful ingredients of plants, it is the group that most interests the pharmaceutical industry. Morphine, strychnine, pilocarpine, atropine and ephedrine drugs are all alkaloids. It is a diverse group, with such a range of characteristics that only generalizations about their composition and actions can be made. The safest such statements are that alkaloids are derived from amino acids and have nitrogen-hydrogen groups (also called amino) in their formulae, they have dramatic effects on the body, and that their function in plants remains a puzzle with most learned opinion suggesting they protect plants from being eaten by all kinds of predators.

Alkaloids do have dramatic actions, many of which are harnessed as medicines. This does not mean they are all toxic and that any plant that contains alkaloids should be shunned or better still banned. It is worth remembering that the stimulant action of tea and coffee comes from several alkaloids and that the white latex in the leaves and stems of .lettuce contains alkaloids (see below).

They are divided into families based· on common chemical structures. Important families are the pyrollizidine alkaloids in borage, ragwort and comfrey; the indole alkaloids, which include the adrenaline and serotonin produced in animals, the harm an of passion flower, reserpine, and the hallucinogenic substances in 'magic mushrooms' *(Psilocybe* mushrooms); the isoquinolines, represented by mescaline, papaverine, nicotine, morphine; and the purine alkaloids, also known as the xanthines, from tea and coffee, which include caffeine, theobromine and theophylline.

Actions of Herbs

Herbalists normally choose herbs for prescriptions on the basis of their actions on the body, and not because they match the patient's symptoms. The symptoms reported by the patient together with the signs seen by the herbalist help to reach a diagnosis. The diagnosis is then interpreted in terms of its causes, and herb actions to bear on these causes are the focus of the prescription. For example, constipation may be treated with herbs that stimulate liver action and bile production; eczema may be treated with herbs that affect the blood and elimination process rather than only to reduce the redness and itching of the rash.

This approach appears alien to non-herbalists who are used to thinking of medicines more symptomatically - a pain reliever for a headache, antacids for indigestion, and even antibiotics for every infection.

Among the main therapeutic actions available to herbalists are important subtleties between herbs. For example, oak bark is a very strong astringent herb but there are milder degrees of astringency from tormentil *(Potentilla erecta)* to ribwort *(Plantago lanceolata)*. Along with these degrees of each action, most herbs offer several different actions, which allows very subtle combinations to be chosen for the specific needs of individual patients.

The main healing actions available to herbalists include the following.

BITTERS

Bitters target the liver and digestive processes and hence are central to many treatment strategies. The liver has a defensible right to the title of 'most important organ in the body'. It is closely involved in the formation of essential substances like proteins, the breakdown of waste for elimination, control of the balance between stored and circulating sugars, and the storage of vital substances like iron and fat-soluble vitamins. The digestive system is also of greater importance than is often allowed for. It must be functioning efficiently for the body to absorb and use the nutrients needed for life, and to dispose of waste products through the bowels and kidneys.

Bitters, not surprisingly, taste bitter. They must do so to work. (See the section above on 'Bitter Principles'.) If the bitterness is disguised by sugar or other substances, the beneficial effects no longer occur.

Bitters may be used in liver or gall bladder conditions where function is reduced; in weakened or sluggish digestion; in constipation due to debility of sluggish digestion; in diabetes; in chronic conditions involving the immune system. They are such good stimulants of digestion in general that they are often used in small amounts in any 'tonic' prescription.

The classic bitter herbs are gentian *(Gentiana lusea)* and centaury *(Centuarium erythraea)*. The thistle family provides bitters which also have particularly beneficial effects on the liver.

Bitters may be good stimulants of liver function (dandelion, *Taraxacum officiruzJe)*, or stimulants of the repair of liver cells damaged by various types of hepatitis (Milk thistle, *Cardus marianus)*. Bitter herbs that are useful for their focus on the stomach secretions and function are horehound *(Marrubium vulgare)*, angelica *(Angelica archangelica)*, wormwood *(Artemisia absinthium)* and its relatives, together with hops *(Humulus luPulus)*.

Most of the bitters focused on the liver stimulate the production of bile in the liver and its movement into the gall bladder for storage. The secretion of bile into the intestines from the gall bladder reservoir is stimulated by mountain grape *(Berberis aquifolium)* and greater celandine *(Chelidonium majus)*.

STIMULANTS

The conventional notion of stimulants as substances that keep people wide awake and possibly with a rush of energy is very different from the herbalist's perspective. Herbal stimulants are used to increase the body's normal functions and are usually targeted at specific organs or activities rather than the whole body. Thus there are general stimulants like kola *(Cola vera)* and mate *(Ilex paraguariensis)* and even coffee as well as circulatory stimulants like chilli *(Capsicum minimum)*, ginger *(Zingiber offiC£,ruz]e)* and prickly ash *(Zanthoxylum americanum)*. Stimulants of the nervous system include the culinary herb rosemary and basil.

Both the digestive and reproductive systems can be stimulated into increased action, The bitters (see above) are stimulants of digestive processes. Damiana *(Turnera diffusa)* stimulates production of the male hormone, testosterone, which has the effect of increasing male sexual function. This herb also has a. folk reputation as an aphrodisiac but any such effect is probably due to the hormonal effects combined with a second valuable property: damiana is a valuable antidepressant. It lifts the gloomy spirit in reactive depression, and there is nothing like depression to lower libido. The effect of removing depression on the libido is an uplifting experience, easily interpreted by the beholder as increased potency.

As stimulants increase activity, there is a danger of using them to mask problems or overcome symptoms. Unless the body's reserves of energy are mobilized or increased, stimulants' can be rapidly depleting or exhausting. Ginseng *(Panax ginseng)* is often abused in this way. It is too often bought from health food shops and used without proper diagnosis or plan of treatment. The immediate effect can be very stimulating but unless there is a substantial reserve of energy, the taker usually experiences exhaustion after about two weeks of daily dosing.

Herbalists take care to use stimulants only in the context of a detailed management plan, where energy and stimulated activity are considered together.

SEDATIVE

Any herb that slows the activity of the central nervous system is a sedative. They are used to slow overactivity in the brain in hysteria or anxiety and insomnia, to reduce pain (analgesics) or ease muscle spasm that is caused by nervous overactivity.

Sedatives are used with care by herbalists, as they slow and ultimately reduce the body's driving energy flow. They do sedate the brain and include tranquillizers and painkillers. However, there are circumstances where sedation is a necessary part of treatment to allow the body's healing processes to progress normally.

Opium is the classic herbal sedative but is no longer available. Useful sedatives include hops, valerian *(Valeriana officinalis)*, lemon balm *(Melissa officinalis)*, Jamaican dogwood *(Piscidia erythrina)*, Californian poppy *(Eschscholzia california)*. Chamomile and valerian are also excellent sedatives for the intestines while hawthorn *(Crataegus oxycanthoides)* is an effective sedative for the heart.

RELAXANTS

Closely related to sedatives, these include herbs that calm the muscles and organs of the body. This also involves the nervous system, but the effect is a gentle calming of the whole body and less sedation of the brain. They relax tension in parts of the body such as the intestines in irritable bowel syndrome or the muscular uterus in painful periods. Tissue and organ tension causes problems like migraines, many bowel disorders, and muscular aches. It can also delay healing. Herbalists often use relaxants targeted on specific parts of the body as part of their healing strategy. They often combine muscle and vascular relaxants with circulatory stimulants to heal joint and muscle injuries; or combine digestive relaxants with bitters to stimulate liver activity in intestinal disease.

Cramp bark *(Viburnum opulus)* and valerian are important general relaxants. Plants' with tropane alkaloids provide specific relaxant herbs for the intestines (belladonna, *Atropa belladonna)*, the lungs (thorn apple, *Datura stramonium)*, and the urinary tubules (henbane, *Hyoscyamus niger)*. For direct application on the skin to relax muscle spasms, lobelia *(Lobelia iriflata)* and lavender are widely used.

ANTISPASMODICS

There are many conditions where muscles go into states of excess and prolonged contraction. The resulting spasms can be painful and disruptive to healthy activity or function. A sports injury can produce protective spasm of the large muscles of movement or smaller muscles protecting a joint. The result is not only pain, but delayed healing if free entry of healing blood is restricted. Excess nervous tension can cause spasms in the intestine that may lead to constipation or the irritable bowel syndrome, which affects 40 per cent of the population. The cramping pain that signals the start of a woman's period is often caused by strong contractions and spasm in the smooth muscles of the uterus. In all such conditions herbalists consider appropriate use of antispasmodic herbs, which are effectively relaxants.

TONICS

'I am feeling low in energy - can I have a tonic?', must be the most common question put to herbalists. The general public concept of a tonic is of a stimulant that will have the taker clicking heels in mid-air and skipping out of the clinic. Herbalists see tonics differently.

Healthy tissues have 'tone'. It is similar to a healthy plant where the cells are pumped full of water so they are tight like inflated balloons. Let a plant run out of water and the cells lose their 'tone' or turgor, and the plant collapses or wilts. Healthy human tissues are also slightly tight, or under a state of healthy tension, or in 'tone'. Human 'tone' is controlled as much by nervous stimulation as by efficient metabolic activity. A tonic remedy is one that increases this tone in tissues and organs. The effect is to restore healthier function and the patient should indeed feel better.

A herbal tonic is a mild stimulation to specific areas of the body and herbs are chosen accordingly. They may be nutritive or simply activating the digestive or other systems of the body.

Patients with regular catarrh in the upper respiratory tract or throughout the body might be given mucous membrane tonics; liver tonics stimulate liver function; nervous tonics are used in conditions of nervous debility after an exhaustive illness, in prolonged depression or stress, or in ME (myalgic encephalomyelitis) and post-viral syndromes.

Tonic herbs include golden seal *(Hydrastis canadensis)* for membranes; wild oats and StJohn's wort *(Hypericum perforatum)* for the nervous system; false unicorn root *(Chamaelir{um luteum)* for the ovaries with lady's mantle *(Alchemilla vulgaris)* for the uterus; dandelion or milk thistle for the liver; and horse chestnut *(Aesculus hippocastanum)* for the vascular system.

HYPER/HYPOTENSIVES

Blood pressure is affected by many processes in the body. The causes of raised blood pressure are often unknown: in this case the curious name 'essential hypertension' is applied. A range of herbs can be used to lower or raise blood pressure. Many act on the nervous control of'theheart's activity, on the blood vessels or on the heart itself.
Hawthorn and broom *(Sarothamnus scoparius)* act on the heart muscle. Useful blood pressure lowering herbs include garlic, lime flowers *(Tilia europea),* valerian, and yarrow *(Achillea tnillefolium).*
Warning: no attempt to treat blood pressure should be made without advice from a qualified herbalist or doctor.

DIURETICS

Diuretics increase the flow of urine. This is helpful in heart conditions where a weakened heart has insufficient pressure to operate the kidney, or when either excessive accumulation of soluble matter in the blood or reduced kidney function leads to the accumulation of water in the blood and body tissues.
The most effective and safe diuretic is dandelion leaf. Others include parsley, coffee, silver birch *(Betula alba),* parsley piert *(Aphanes arvensis),* and pellitory-of-the-wall *(Parietaria diffusa).*

CARDIOACTIVES

Many people are surprised at the value of herbal remedies in heart disease. Apart from the importance of garlic in reducing cholesterol, blood clotting and blood pressure, herbs that act directly on the heart muscle are valuable in any herbalist's practice. The foxglove *(Digitalis purpurea)* was used by herbalists long before the heart drug digoxin was extracted. Digoxin is called a cardioactive glycoside. Other useful plants also contain these glycosides or other substances that also have an action on the heart. Arterial disease, high and low blood pressure, arrhythmias and heart failure can all be treated with herbal medicines that have appropriate action on the heart. All heart diseases should be treated only by a qualified herbalist or doctor.
Cardioactive herbs include hawthorn *(Crataegus oxycanthoides)*, Lily-of-the-valley *(Corwallaria maJalis)*, squill *(Urginea man'tima)*, broom *(Sarothamnun scoparius)*, ephedra *(Ephedra sinica)*, and motherwort *(Leonorus cardiaca)*.

STYPTICS AND HAEMOSTATICS

Both these actions stop the excess loss of blood from bleeding.
Astringents are applied externally to stop wounds bleeding. Internal bleeding is treated with herbs like horsetail, plantain, yarrow, or shepherd's purse *(Capsella bursa-pastoris)*.

LAXATIVES

Herbalists are always interested in the nature and frequency of bowel activity, because of the importance of waste elimination to good health. The indigestible contents of the diet and the action of bile salts on the intestine encourage efficient bowel actions in healthy people. Occasionally, laxative support may be necessary.

There are three types of laxatives. Stimulant laxatives increase the motility of the bowel, which increases the rate of movement of the stool through the bowel. Osmotic laxatives increase the amount of water held in the stool as it passes through the bowel, thus helping keep the stool large and soft so it passes along and out easily. Bulk laxatives provide large amounts of indigestible matter, which ensures that stools have bulk so there is something for the bowel muscles to work on and to pass through the bowel. Herbs are available for each laxative action.

Stimulant laxatives can be bought freely in chemists and are overused. They are normally taken long before they are necessary and their overuse makes the bowel so lazy that the natural bowel-emptying actions are lost and laxatives become essential through habituation. Herbalists use laxatives only when necessary and then for the shortest possible time. Careful choice of diet and maintaining a healthy, active digestive system are the best ways of ensuring laxatives are not needed regularly.

Laxative herbs range from the bulk laxatives like psyllium or flea seed *(Plantago ovata)* , through gentle stimulants like yellow dock *(Rumex crispus)* and senna *(Cassia senna)*, to strong purgatives like cascara *(Rhamnus purshiana)* and alder buckthorn *(Rhamnus frangula)*. Many liver herbs tend to have a laxative effect through their action on the bile. Small amounts of dandelion in a prescription are often sufficient to make the bowel more regular and the stool softer.

EMETICS

These cause vomiting which is a drastic but occasionally necessary form of elimination. Most emetics stimulate the lining of the stomach. Lobelia and ipecacuanha or ipecac are the two notable emetics but many expectorants are emetic in larger doses. Ipecac is used in orthodox medicine for the same purpose.

ANTI EMETICS

Travel sickness, morning sickness in pregnancy, anxiety, migraine and even overindulgence in food can produce feelings of nausea or lead to vomiting. Black horehound *(Ballota nigra)*, peppermint, ginger and chamomile suppress the feeling of sickness. Chamomile should be tried beforehand, as some people do not like the taste or smell of the herb and can be made nauseous by drinking it.

CARMINATIVES

These calm the digestive tract by relieving flatulence (wind) and the painful colic that comes with it. Helpful herbs are generally those rich in volatile oils and include many kitchen herbs and spices. Asian spices including cumin, coriander, fennel, cinnamon and cardamom are very useful. Peppermint and chamomile teas taken after meals are also effective.

ANTIMICROBIALS, ANTISEPTICS ETC.

There are many different ways of keeping pathogenic organisms at bay. Antibiotics are usually derived from fungi or bacteria, and are used against bacteria. Antivirals destroy viruses. An antimicrobial substance destroys a wide range of organisms, including fungi, bacteria, viruses etc. An antiseptic prevents infections and is usually applied to the skin and not taken internally.

The herbal repertoire is well stocked with herbs against a whole range of organisms. Many herbs are antiseptic and antimicrobial. Sage, garlic, thyme, wild indigo *(Baptisia tinctoria)* and myrrh *(Commiplwra molmol)* are notable examples. Fungi are attacked by tea tree oil, marigold *(Calendula officina/ is)*, and thyme.

Echinacea, lemon balm oil *(Melissa officinalis)*, and marigold are particularly effective against viruses. Intestinal worms are held at bay with garlic, thyme and tansy.

ANTI-INFECTIVE

The antimicrobials etc. above act directly on the pathogenic organism and either kill it or make its growth and reproduction impossible. Herbalists have another strategy against infections of all types. They have herbs that can stimulate the immune system, which is 'normally responsible for tracking down and attacking any foreign organisms that enter the tissues or blood. .

The white blood cells in particular are active protectors against infection. Echinacea and Shiitake mushroom have a particular reputation for boosting a weakened immune system and so helping to fight off infection.

ANTITUSSIVES AND EXPECTORANTS

Coughs are the body's way of expelling unwanted substances from the throat and lungs, whether it be heavy mucus during a lung infection or the accumulated dust and grime from breathing in dirty air. Such coughs should be encouraged, as they are cleansing. However, there can be coughs that are due to irritations of the throat and larynx and these can be very frustrating. Here an antitussive can help switch off the cough reflex and save further irritation from dry coughing. Expectorants help soften and dislodge phlegm or catarrh from the lungs and throat. An expectorant needs the cough to expel the catarrh so it is useless, as often happens with pharmaceutical

'cough medicines', to combine an expectorant with an antitussive. Herbalists have different types of expectorants available. There are relaxing expectorants for tight spastic conditions like asthma and bronchitis, and stimulating expectorants for use in heavy infective chests where congestion is normal.

Most expectorants work by reflex action following their action on the stomach lining. Some work by stimulating the natural hairs, or cilia, in the tubes within the lung to carry particles of dust and mucus up to the top of the bronchi where they can be swallowed or coughed up more easily. Others work by soothing bronchial spasm and softening the phlegm clinging to the small tubules deep within the lungs. Relaxing expectorants include coltsfoot *(Tussilago farfara),* .ribwort *(Plantago lanceolata),* thyme, liquorice, hyssop *(Hyssopus officinalis).* Stimulating expectorants include elecampane *(Inula helenium),* cowslip *(Primula veris),* and squill *(Urginia man·tima).* Expectorants like thyme and hyssop combine useful antimicrobial activity with their expectorant quality.

ANTICATARRHAL

Mucus (catarrh or phlegm) is the well-known secretion from the mucous membranes of the respiratory tract. The stuffy nose in a cold or sinusitis and the seemingly immovable blob at the back of the throat, which causes the repeated attempts at clearing the throat, are often due to catarrh. The causes are legion. In colds, it is from membrane irritation by a virus infection. In hypersensitivity states, irritation from passing particles that cause local inflammation are responsible. Smokers cough regularly due to the direct irritation from the smoke in the lungs and indirectly due to the need to remove mucus oozing from the inflamed and irritated lung membranes. Many people tend to have more general catarrh. They are constantly cold, relatively inactive and have a tendency to long periods of thin or watery mucus in their nose and throat. This state is metabolic and is often made worse by foods like dairy products and bread. They often have congested and catarrhal mucous membranes in other parts of their body, including the intestines and urinary tracts.

Herbal treatment is broad-based, with diet change as necessary and mixtures of circulation and eliminative remedies combined with specific remedies against catarrh. Astringent herbs like ground ivy *(Glechwma hederacea)*, ribwort, golden seal, elder flowers *(Sambucus nigra)* and golden rod *(Solidago virgaurea)* are standards,

DIAPHORETICS

An infection is often accompanied naturally by a fever. This rise in body temperature and sweating is part of the natural defence against invasion by foreign organisms. It is usually a mistake to suppress the slight fever of minor colds and even flu because healing is delayed. Herbalists often manage the natural fever reaction by using herbs that can cause a rise in body temperature and sweating, which simulates and helps control a natural fever. The herbs used are called diaphoretics. They cause a feeling of flushing and lead to perspiration.

Useful remedies include elder flower, yarrow, peppermint and ginger.

ANTI·INFLAMMATORY

Inflammation is a natural and healthy process - most of the time. The redness around a minor burn, insect bite or infected cut is a visible sign of the protective inflammatory process. It is the body's reaction to infection, injury or irritation. It causes dilation of local blood vessels and an increased flow of blood and other fluid to the affected area, which explains the redness.

Special bacteria-destroying blood cells enter injured tissue and the increased flow of blood into an area speeds injury or wound healing. Inflamed areas are thus usually swollen (from increased inflow of blood and other fluids), red (from increased blood flow), hot (from both the increased metabolic activity of healing and the increased blood flow), and painful (from the pressure of the swelling).

Herbalists see inflammation as evidence that the body's defence and repair mechanisms are working well. Inflammation is usually welcomed and watched to gauge the speed with which the body heals itself. But sometimes the underlying cause of the inflammation persists and the inflammation itself becomes a problem. Anyone who has experienced gout in a big toe or the unremitting pain of rheumatic joints knows the pain of this healthy process. Other chronic inflammatory conditions include diverticulosis, Crohn's disease, bronchitis and eczema. ' This excess or chronic inflammation is approached by herbalists with relief for the symptoms, and also active measures to reduce the underlying cause. Many herbs are considered anti-inflammatory and most work to speed the work of the inflammatory process rather than merely suppressing it. Bitters, volatile oils and chemicals called sesquiterpene lactones are found in popular remedies. Wormwood and gentian are two bitter herbs widely used. Other anti-inflammatory are meadowsweet, white willow *(Salix alba)*, devil's claw *(HarpagopJrytum procumbens)*, liquorice, marigold, chamomile, hydrastis, figwort and burdock.

ALTERATIVES

These act on the metabolism, shifting it in a beneficial direction. Alteratives are often linked to the depuratives or 'blood cleansers', as many plants have these actions in common. They are a curious but very useful collection of herbs that work by enhancing the blood's important functions of elimination and protection. They include herbs that act on the lymph system, which is a form of garbage collection system filtering waste materials and bacteria from the fluids which bathe all cells in the body, and dumping them in the blood for elimination through action of the liver and kidneys.

Herbalists use alteratives in tissue congestive states or where there is an impaired immune system. Conditions include skin complaints like eczema and psoriasis, joint inflammations, swollen lymph glands, chronic infective states, and tumours. Herbs include echinacea, burdock, cleavers *(Galium apan'ne)*, heartsease, yellow dock *(Rumex crispus)*, and poke root *(PJrytolacca decandra)*.

UTERINE AND MENSTRUAL

This group incorporates many actions directed specifically at conditions of the uterus and associated organs and tissues. The emmenagogues, which stimulate menstrual flow, are essentially abortifacients (abortion-inducing) and are used with great care by professional herbalists. Many herbs, even common culinary herbs, have this action to some degree and it is important for any pregnant woman to consult a herbalist before treating herself with any herbal medicines. While some uterine conditions do require stimulation, herbalists as often are looking to tone or relax uterine tissues and choose from a wide range of relevant herbs.

Many menstrual problems, including painful periods, excess flow, irregular periods, premenstrual syndrome (PMS or PMT), mid-cycle bleeding, cessation of periods, endometriosis and symptoms of menopause respond to herbal remedies.

Many other gynaecological conditions, such as infections, inflammation (including pelvic inflammatory disease), infertility and hormonal imbalances are treated with herbs offering the relevant actions.

Uterine herbs include lady's mantle, guelder rose, motherwort, blue cohosh *(Caulophyllum thalictroides)*, pasque flower *(Anemone pulsatilla)*, squaw vine *(Mitchella repens)*, helonias root or false unicorn root *(Chamaelerium luteum)*, white dead nettle *(Lamium album)*, and raspberry leaf. See also Hormonal herbs below.

HORMONAL

There are many health problems associated with either over-
or underactive endocrine glands - glands that secrete
essential hormones into the bloodstream. These glands
include the pituitary, thyroid, adrenals, ovaries, testicles and
pancreas.
Herbalists have access to an armoury of herbs that have
dramatic or subtle effects on selected glands and thus
influence the hormonal output and balance of the body.
Many such herbs contain steroidal saponins which closely
resemble the chemical structure of human hormones. Herbs
include vitex or chaste berry, sarsaparilla, liquorice, wild yam,
and saw palmetto *(Serenoa semdata)*, and both Siberian and
Asian ginsengs.

WOUND HEALERS

The formal name for this action is vulnerary. Many actions
may be drawn up to heal different types of wounds. Weeping
burns or bleeding wounds may be treated with strong
astringents like oak bark or comfrey leaf, which form a
protective coat stopping the loss of fluid or blood and
keeping infective organisms out.
The tannins in astringents have the additional benefit of
being antiseptic. Heavy mucilages, such as are found in
comfrey, shrink on drying and help pull the edges of open
wounds together. Comfrey also contains an interesting
chemical, alantoin, which promotes the regeneration of
connective tissue and thus speeds the rate of healing in the
protected wound.
Other wound-healing herbs include many of the astringents,
and marigold, St John's Wort, chamomile, arnica or witch
hazel.

DEMULCENTS AND EMOLLIENTS

These actions sooth and soften surfaces to which they are applied. They are useful to protect irritated or inflamed membranes like the throat, stomach or urinary tract and help reduce the irritation of eczema and related skin conditions. Classic herbs are rich in mucilages or saponins and include comfrey, marshmallow, slippery elm, liquorice, flea seed *(Psyllium ovata)* , plantain and coltsfoot.

ANTIPRURITIC

Itching (pruritis) is one of the most annoying symptoms and often demands instant relief. Many conditions, from liver disease through eczema and urticaria to persistent anal itch, are recognizable. Causes are variable and herbalists direct their selection of treatment to appropriate actions but chickweed is the outstanding herb for relieving the itch while other herbs do the healing.

ANODYNE (PA1N RELIEF)

Pain relief is often necessary symptom relief. Headaches can be relieved by betony *(Stacl!Js betonica)* or feverfew (*Tanacetum parthenium)* depending on the cause. Colicky or spastic intestinal pains may be approached with antispasmodics like belladonna. joint pain responds to anti-inflammatories like devil's claw or others with analgesic ingredients like white willow. The strongest herbal painkillers contain alkaloids and include Californian poppy, Jamaican dogwood, gelsemium and aconite. Warning: strong herbal painkillers are potentially dangerous and should be used only on the advice of a qualified herbalist.

ANTHELMINTICS (ANTIWORM)

Intestinal worms are common, especially among young schoolchildren. Herbs that destroy infestations include garlic, tansy, wormwood, and thyme. Different worms require different herbs so it is best to consult a herbalist to identify the culprits before starting treatment.

Chapter Six

Are Herbal Medicines Safe?

Consider the typical Western diet. It contains many plant foods: cereals, pulses, root and leaf vegetables, fruits of enormous variety, not to forget the myriad of seeds, barks, leaves and fruits that are used as culinary herbs and spices. Are these safe? Take an idyllic English country-cottage garden. Envisage the hollyhocks, aconites and the lilac tree by the back door. In a true cottage garden, there will be numerous wildflowers, including belladonna, cuckoopint and, under the weeping branches of the beech trees, several beautiful fly agaric mushrooms. Is a garden safe? Clearly the answer depends. It depends on what is meant by 'safe'. Most people take 'safe' here to mean that no unexpected harm should result. It is usually meant as an absolute concept.

Thus eating bread, the staff of life, should bring pleasure and important nutrients, but is not expected to be in any way harmful. Bread is thought of as 'safe' because nobody expects, even as a remote risk, that eating bread might cause damage to their liver or permanent brain damage. Most people would also, classify beer as a 'safe' drink because the desired intoxication from drinking it should come without any real risk of bacterial poisoning or being infected by typhoid. The fact that the alcohol in beer damages the liver and brain, both of which can and do cause serious illness and death, does not make beer 'unsafe' in daily conversation. It makes the *drinking of too much beer* unsafe to health.

There is also the matter of relative safety and how the true measure of risk is calculated, estimated, or given importance by individuals. The real chances of dying from smoking or alcohol-related illness are far greater than dying from food additives, and yet many people show greater concern for the action of additives than for that of smoking or drinking. Many people also dismiss or ignore real risks to their health by choice and thus distort the real dangers. The classic is the cigarette-smoking, bottle-of-wine-a-day gastronome who scoffs an artery-clogging diet of cream sauces and animal fat, but refuses to drink the city's tap water because it contains nitrates that might cause cancer one day. One person's health risk is another's pastime.

It is the nature of the risk to health, and not only the size of the risk that matters. Eating too much of any member of the melon family of plants (including cucumbers) is almost certain to cause indigestion. That is a high risk of a minor problem.

However, the chances of getting aflatoxin poisoning from eating food-grade peanuts in Britain is extremely unlikely, though it is serious when it occurs. The result is a damaged liver at best or death for the less lucky.

When talking about the safety of drugs, herbal or not, there are two main types of problem. First are minor unwanted effects that can occur in any patient taking a drug at the prescribed dose. These are effects that occur in addition to the planned therapeutic effect. Pharmacologists who study the action and effects of medicinal drugs state that any substance possessing therapeutic effects must also have unwanted effects. These may be severe, even life-threatening, or be unnoticeable. This seems to be a fact of biochemistry and there is no reason to believe that herbs are different. Minor unwanted effects are called side effects and include nausea, loose bowels, a drop in blood pressure, or headache (see below). The more serious unwanted effects are the real concern with safety. They are called adverse or toxic effects and include serious illness or discomfort from taking the drug as prescribed.

With pharmaceutical drugs, adverse effects account for 5 out of every 100 occupied hospital beds and are reported in up to 20 per cent of all patients while in hospital. The effects include blood disorders, hepatitis, adrenal failure, heart problems, and internal bleeding. The most common drug culprits in deaths from adverse reactions are digoxin or digitoxin, antibiotics, aspirin, steroids, anticoagulants and phenylbutazone (a strong anti-inflammatory used in hospitals). The true extent of adverse reactions is unknown because few doctors willingly admit to causing harm to patients by their treatments and such effects are under-reported. Such a high toll from modern drugs is not unexpected. They are increasingly strong drugs and, as their number and chemical complexity increases, the likelihood of straightforward effects increases and the risks are added to by the chances of interactions between different drugs being taken at the same time. Even diligent doctors have an impossible task keeping up with the risks to their patients from new drugs.

Safety must be kept clearly in perspective, as the following discussion .about our daily food reminds.

Safety in Foods and Garden Plants

Many common foods are poisonous. Peanuts are often contaminated by fungi that produce poisonous chemicals called aflatoxins, which seriously damage the liver. Peanut oil itself contains a fatty acid, behenic acid, that damages blood vessels and so perhaps even peanut butter could be considered unsafe. Apple and apricot seeds contain cyanides. Nutmeg is hallucinogenic. Many foods cause dangerous sensitivity reactions, including angioedema, where the tissues of the throat and nose swell quickly, which can restrict breathing and even be fatal. Peanuts and lychee can cause angioedema.

Anaphylactic shock, which can be fatal, can follow eating mangoes, strawberries and oranges. There is also the catalogue of safety hazards from natural carcinogens in foods, food poisoning from bacterial contaminants during storage or preparation of foods, pesticides applied during cultivation or storage of foods, and of course, from the many additives used in the preparation and manufacture of most food in industrial societies. Food can be bad for health. Gardens contain many poisonous plants. Children die from eating laburnum seeds, belladonna berries or the beautiful monkshood. Older and wiser people are made very ill, or even die, from incompetently experimenting with wild mushrooms, 'mistaking hemlock for parsley, or using meadow saffron instead of the commercial colouring. Many common wild plants are poisonous: hellebores and spurges, columbine, privet hedges, buttercup, ivy, mistletoe, dog's mercury, foxglove, and yew.

The central matter is the question of dose. Many foods are unsafe in small or normal daily doses. Carcinogens, and foods producing sensitivity reactions, need be eaten only in small amounts. Pesticides and additives usually need to be eaten in larger amounts, but not so large they are impossible to consume.

In fact, many additives and pesticides used on foods are approved by governments in the full knowledge of their potential for damaging health. Usually they are assumed to be 'safe enough' because the amount of food that would have to be consumed before 'unacceptable harm' occurred is thought to be greater than 'reasonable average consumption'. The same dose caveat applies to garden plants. While a mouthful of yellow stainer mushroom or henbane can kill, an adult would have to consume several handfuls of their privet hedge before serious illness might occur. Such a feat of consumption would be expected only in the very determined masochist. Most garden or wild plants need to be eaten in significant amounts before any serious harm would be expected.

Safety of Herbal Medicines

What about herbal medicines? Taking herbal medicines prescribed by a qualified practitioner is as safe as eating normal foods. Taking commonly available herbal preparations like herb teas, dandelion leaves in salads and so on, is also as safe as eating a fruit and vegetable diet.

Many herbal medicines are otherwise used daily as foods: garlic, sage, thyme, pepper, ginger, etc. The majority of the others are not known to be harmful, even though they may be from local wild plants or imported from other countries. Remember the history of herbal remedies. Just as the thousands of years of experience with the healing properties was noted,

selected and passed on to succeeding generations, the same vigilance would have been applied to poisonous herbs. It is difficult to imagine how any plant showing poisonous properties at therapeutic doses could have been passed on, even when it also had desired medicinal qualities.

A minority of medicinal herbs are potentially toxic. These are plants whose active ingredients are 'strong' chemicals with pronounced effects on the body. The particular effects displayed give these plants their specific medicinal importance. These plants include solanaceous plants - belladonna, thorn apple, and henbane - containing valuable tropane alkaloids. Aconite contains a powerful sedative and is used for intractable nerve pains like trigeminal neuralgia. The plants containing strongly cardio active ingredients are also, not surprisingly, included among the herbs to be respected. These valuable herbs are well understood and respected by the practitioner, who has been trained in their use. Most are Scheduled Poisons, which herbalists are allowed to use under the Medicines Act, 1968.Not only can they be used only by herbalists, but their dosage is strictly controlled by law. Thus, where herbs are known to have powerful properties, they are respected and their use is strictly controlled within the profession.

Warning: it is obvious that nobody other than a qualified practitioner should attempt to prepare or give any medicine prepared from these plants, even though they may be. Found growing freely in the wild.

Recent scares in the media have focused on two possible serious effects from herbs, liver damage and cancer. There is a theoretical mechanism for substances in herbs to irritate the liver, just as pharmaceutical drugs often do. However, there are no reported instances in the UK of liver damage being unequivocally attributed to medicinal herbs. In 1989, two letters in the *British Medical journal* suggested that two patients, who had developed mild hepatitis, were suffering the effects of herbal products containing valerian and scutellaria. The letters merely raised the suggestion, but it led to a minor scare in the press.

Closer examination showed that only the loosest of connections could be made and, in one case, the formulation of the bought product had been changed six months prior to it being purchased. The supposed harmful herbs had not been in the product taken by the ill woman. Subsequently, the authors wrote again emphasizing they were not saying the herbs *caused* the hepatitis, only that all doctors should ask their patients what herbal drugs they are taking. At the time, there were over 30 million doses of the offending products, Kalms and Neurolax, being taken each year in the UK without any report of harm. Nor have there been subsequent reports of proven harm, despite the publicity given in Britain.

More recently, doctors at London's Great Ormond Street Hospital for sick children began research with Chinese herbs in the treatment of childhood eczema. They were using the herbs in children so sick that they were confined to hospital where they would normally be covered from head to toe in hydrocortisone cream to relieve the terrible itch of their eczema. At the start of the research the doctors didn't know the identity of the herbs in the prescription, much less their ingredients. As research progressed, doctors were monitoring not only the improvement in the eczema but also the effects of the herbs on the children's livers and general health. They have found no sign of harm to the children.

Side Effects and Safety Record of Herbal Medicine

Experience with herbs has shown very few noticeable side effects. Practitioners tend to check with patients on both the benefits of their treatment and any side effects. Most herbs in regular clinical use are well tolerated by patients and usually no side effects are reported at all. The most common side effects are limited to headache, nausea and looseness of the bowels.

Other less common side effects include skin rashes in people known to be sensitive to salicylates with herbs like meadow sweet, and increased blood pressure with long treatment with liquorice. Herbalists know of such effects and monitor patients closely, reducing dosage or altering the prescription if such effects appear.

There are several good reasons why herbal medicines tend to be so safe. The complex mixture of chemical constituents of plants includes substances like the tannins and saponins which tend to moderate the activity of the more active chemicals. This is the effect of the total action of the mixture of plant ingredients being very different from the action of isolated or concentrated chemicals. In addition, the way herbal medicines are used means that the amount of each ingredient in a dose is very small compared to the dosages in pharmaceutical medicines. Thus, the risk from even the more active chemicals in plants is smaller.

Dose is also important. While a plant might not be safe in large doses, the doses used by herbalists are low enough that any theoretical harmful effect is not experienced. In technical terms, this means that there is a wide gap between the therapeutic dose of most herbs and the dose at which side effects or toxicity are expected, thus making herbs safe medicines.

But a more important reason lies in the combination of how herbal remedies were selected over the centuries and their therapeutic actions in the body. Just as Darwinian selection of genes in evolution tended towards selection of the fittest, the way remedies were selected throughout history identified the safest and most effective herbs, as explained above. Thus the handed down remedies tend to be the safer plants from the tens of thousands of possible plants that grow around us. In addition, medicinal herbs are used because of their actions in *encouraging normal body functions* and it would be contradictory if a medicinal herb were to encourage any toxic reaction. That is not to say there are not strong, even potentially toxic herbs; rather that herbs are chosen and used to encourage healthier functioning and not, like pharmaceutical drugs, to suppress symptoms or block the function of overactive organs. Herb remedies are thus less likely to be chosen from among plants known to have toxic effects at therapeutic doses.

The safety of herbs should also be compared with the safety of pharmaceutical drugs, which many people are choosing to avoid because of concerns' over safety and side effects. The horrors of unsafe drugs like Thalidomide and Opren may be extremes, but are still being discovered only after drugs have been licensed and used on thousands of patients. In the 1980s,

Professor Michael Oliver, then President of the British Cardiac Society, wrote a leading article in the *Lancet*, asking colleagues why the new beta-blocker drug propanalol was being prescribed so freely when so little was known about its action, benefits or safety. Serious illness like hepatitis, for example, is a common consequence of many prescribed drugs and is viewed by the medical profession as normal and expected. Mothers are told to accept the risk of brain, damage from whooping cough vaccination as an acceptable cost of the benefits of avoiding the illness. Even very common drugs that can be bought over the counter by children are relatively unsafe. The most used painkillers in Britain, aspirin and paracetamol, are responsible for over 100deaths each year; aspirin from internal bleeding and paracetamol from liver damage. It is surely unacceptable that such risks from pharmaceutical drugs are expected; but it is outrageous that they are seen as a *normal* consequence of drug treatment. Little wonder such energies go into attempts to discredit the safer herbal medicines.

Safe herbs are not necessarily safe for all people. The same applies for all types of drugs. Pregnant women are vulnerable to herbs that have stimulating effects on the uterus, even though the same herbs may be specifically indicated for certain conditions in non-pregnant women. People suffering from conditions like inflamed kidneys or high blood pressure would obviously not be given herbs containing volatile oils or herbs that may raise blood pressure respectively. Children under two years old would not be given herbs that placed any great demands on the metabolism.

There is a tendency in some sections of the media to get overexcited about the safety of herbal medicines. Occasionally there are sensible warnings about keeping children away from poisonous garden plants. But most alarms are either the results of misinformation or appear to be carefully-orchestrated attempts by elements in the orthodox medical profession or pharmaceutical industry to discredit herbal medicines. The

American Food and Drug Administration decided that the popular American tea, sassafras, was unsafe on the grounds that it contained an alkaloid which, when isolated and concentrated, could cause cancer in rats. Neither the fact that the alkaloid was insoluble in water, and thus didn't appear in the tea, nor the failure to produce any evidence of a single human liver cancer caused by the tea, even after 200 years of experience, seemed to influence their decision.

The American Medical Association (AMA) began a campaign against herbal teas in the late 1970s. Part of the strategy seemed to be based on the notion of blaming so many common herbal teas with health risks that herbs in general would be suspected by the population. They were inept in concept and execution. One of their claims was that chamomile tea caused anaphylactic shock. However, they failed to follow one of the fundamental requirements of scientific inquiry, namely, to gather supporting evidence. As doctors could find only a single example of chamomile-induced anaphylaxis in any medical literature as far back into the archives as 1850.

Assuming that was a genuine case, it remained at least a rare phenomenon if not a unique one.

Shortly after the rumblings in the American literature, the respected British newspaper, the *Independent,* published an article with the headline 'Beware the herbs that harm as well as heal', a mirror image of the American statements about the 'potential harm' from herbal medicines without giving any evidence of that harm and, of course, without any comparison of the harm from pharmaceutical drugs. The British Consumers' Association also leapt onto the rickety bandwagon with a well publicized report titled 'Kill or cure'. The horrors awaiting the gardener included chamomile, which was included in a table of 'potentially harmful remedies'. The reason? It is claimed to cause skin rashes, although they didn't get around to offering any evidence on how often or how severe.

Chamomile tea must be one of the two or three most popular herbal teas in Europe. Surely such effects would be reported more often if they were real or significant? They might have included cabbages, which cause mouth ulcers, and strawberries, which cause hypersensitivity rashes in about 15 per cent of people (though I wouldn't call either effect 'harmful').

A more reasoned, scientific view of the safety of herbal medicines recognizes them as 'safe' in the commonly accepted sense and as 'safer' in general than their pharmaceutical alternatives. Much of the enduring popularity of herbal medicines among the public comes from awareness of the safety of herbs when compared with other drug alternatives and their effectiveness. Herbal medicines are drugs and so should be treated with the same respect as any drug. They should be used only as indicated and at the recommended doses. While efforts to discredit herbs will continue, the important information to keep asking for, to look for in each accusation, and to evaluate carefully is the *evidence* that herbs are harmful.

It is most curious that scientifically based bodies like the medical profession, the pharmaceutical industry, and the food and drug regulation bodies in all industrial countries continue to attack the safety of herbs without offering evidence of the harm.

Innuendo is easier and can be more subversive. What worries them most - that their best available evidence against herbs will not stand scrutiny, or that whatever evidence is available will allow direct comparison with the harm from orthodox medicines, and show herbal remedies in an even better light?

Chapter Seven

Case Histories

Every patient is different. Herbalists don't treat cases of rheumatism or eczema; they treat *people* who have symptoms of these or other conditions. The following brief case histories show how herbalists approach common problems and explain both the general management of the patients and their herbal treatments. These histories come from my own experience and reflect my approach to each patient and their condition. No two herbalists could be expected to treat the same patient in an identical manner, but their basic approach should be the same.

Note: The herbal treatments included with the histories should not be used for any patient with the same diagnosis or even similar symptoms. Each prescription is designed for that individual patient.

Premenstrual Syndrome (PMS)/
Premenstrual Tension (PMT)

Sally was 34 years old. She had two children (10 and 12 years old) and had lived with her partner for 15 years. Before her children were born, her periods had been regular (28 day cycle), would last 3-5 days with some tolerable spasmodic pain on the first day, but without any significant PMT symptoms. On many occasions the first warning of her periods was the cramping pain on day one. Shortly after the first child she noticed she was becoming tearful, depressed and irritable for up to a week before her periods. Sometimes she became so irritable that she felt guilty for the effect it had on her children and partner. Bloating and water retention added to her misery.

Sally was otherwise healthy. Her bowel function was passable but she experienced occasional constipation and stools tended to be firmer than comfort would like. She had a busy life, perhaps working too hard with her job as editor with a publisher and trying to look after both young children and the house when she got home. Her partner helped, but this did not diminish the feeling of responsibility nor the sheer volume of household work.

Exercise had slipped into history since she left school. Eating at work was dominated by office coffee and chocolate bats.

Home meals were better but her diet was too full of microwave meals while fresh salads, vegetables or fruit were seen only every second day or so.

HERBAL APPROACH

Sally has classic symptoms of PMT, together with aggravating factors including the stressful lifestyle, coffee and chocolate, and reduced exercise. Her diet needs improvement to increase the 'cleansing' components of fruit and fresh vegetables and shift the bowel to better regularity. Chocolate and coffee should be dropped from the diet.

The herbal prescription aimed to rebalance the ovarian hormones (oestrogen and progesterone) with vitex, tone the uterus and especially the ovaries with helonias root, and discourage water retention with a diuretic. To help reduce pressure on the nervous system, the gentle nervous trophorestorative and anxiety reliever skullcap was added.

HERBAL PRESCRIPTION		
Helonias root	*Chamaelirium luteum*	20 ml
Dandelion leaf	*Taraxacum officinale*	30 ml
Vitex	*folia*	20 ml
Skullcap	*Vitex agnus-castus*	30 ml
	Scutellaria laterifolia	100 ml
Dose: 5 ml three times daily in water.		

After the first month, her period was three days early, which is common with vitex treatment and the bloating and breast tenderness, were less. By the third month, periods were regular and PMT symptoms had reduced by about 80 per cent. Water retention was barely noticeable and the most important symptom for Sally, the irritability, had gone. After three months, medication was reduced to only 20 drops of vitex each morning for the second 14 days of Sally's cycle. This was continued for the next three months then stopped.

Over these 3 months, symptoms progressively receded, ending up being less than 20 per cent of the original symptoms.

Fourteen months later, Sally's PMT has remained under control and quite tolerable. Chocolate and coffee have been dropped totally and, together with an improved diet generally, Sally feels much better.

Irritable Bowel Syndrome

Charlie came with complaints of a grumbling stomach, roaming colicky pains, wind and bowel movements that ranged from painful constipation to diarrhoea. He was a 27-year-old computer engineer who had been trying to combine an Evening University course with a promotion that based his future with the company on annual performance assessments. He had suffered from the symptoms for 3 years. He had seen his GP who .examined him and prescribed Fybogel - a pharmaceutical drug based on flea seed husks - which had no effect. His diet was reasonable but meals were irregular and alcohol consumption was high at 24 units a week. He lived with a partner and the relationship seemed happy enough except that there was too little time together because of his work and this brought occasional complaints.

An examination of Charlie's abdomen showed there was tenderness over his lower colon in the left side of the pelvis, where there was also some tension in the wall of the colon on the right side. The sounds in his intestine resembled an approaching tube train instead of the more relaxed, gentle gurgles every 10-15 seconds in a normal gut. There was occasional mucus in the bowel movements but no blood. The diagnosis was irritable bowel precipitated by stress.

HERBAL APPROACH

Irritable bowel is often a statement of healthy reaction to chronic stress. The 'gut is closely linked to the central nervous system and is governed by its own autonomic nerve supply. Stress rapidly disrupts the normal functioning, reducing digestion and gut motility in order to shift blood to the muscles of the arms and legs for the innate 'flight or fight' reaction to stress. The longer the stress continues, the more the gut seems to get locked into this abnormal functioning and IBS results.

The herbal approach to relax the over-toned muscles of the gut, coupled with some stress reduction of the central nervous system to turn off the signals to the gut. This helps relieve symptoms within a week or so, when normal function should start again.

Charlie was encouraged to take up some exercise and to think about how more quality time could be spent with his partner.

A happier home life could mean a happier partner as well as helping to ease the stress of his current lifestyle. Herbal treatment focused on relaxing both Charlie and his gut for three weeks.

HERBAL PRESCRIPTION		
Valerian	*Valeriana officinalis*	40 ml
Chamomile	*Matricaria recutita*	40 ml
Meadowsweet	*Filipendula ulmaria*	20 ml
		100 ml
Dose: 5 ml three times a day in water before meals.		

This prescription was followed for two weeks. His symptoms reduced steadily and he felt more calm and relaxed in himself.

At his second visit (two weeks) the importance of looking to his lifestyle to reduce avoidable stress was made clear and was understood. He had already decided to change employers as soon as his university course finished, and had planned to take an extra year to finish the course to reduce the pressure.

After a further two weeks on the starting prescription, the medication was changed to:

HERBAL PRESCRIPTION		
Chamomile	*Matricaria recutita*	20 ml
Dandelion root	*Taraxacum oJIicinal.e*	30 ml
Golden rod	*radix*	30 ml
Valerian	*Solido.go virgaurea*	20 ml
	Valeriano. officinalis	100 ml
Dose: 5 ml three times a day in water before meals.		

After 6 weeks, symptoms ceased completely and Charlie's irritable bowel and abdomen returned to desirable normality. He did well to tackle stress in his life and is managing the unavoidable stresses with more time devoted to relaxation. He recently took up meditation.

Eczema

Richard was 13. His mother brought him with eczema on his arms, and the backs of his legs. He had this since he was two and, although she had hoped it would disappear by the time he was seven or so, it had persisted and was driving them both to distraction. The rash seemed to vary in intensity from day to day. She had been given hydrocortisone cream by the GP but it seemed only to relieve the rash which soon reappeared.
Richard was pale, irritable, a 'nervy' boy, and occupied himself by scratching his rash. He had a good appetite but had a diet rich in crisps, sweets and cola, just like his school friends.

There was little room for healthy food because his appetite was soon satisfied. The family diet was meat and two veg, with plenty of fried foods, little fruit and lots of milk puddings and cheddar cheese. Richard was not breast fed. His mother had trouble starting in hospital and was moved onto bottle feeding before she left to come home. There were no other children so all the parents' attention and expectations were sitting upon Charlie's shoulders. It seemed there were emotional stresses in the family. Charlie has no history of asthma or hay fever, suggesting he is not an atopic type (genetically likely to develop eczema, asthma or hay fever in childhood).

HERBAL APPROACH

Eczema in children has many causes, but diet and stress often play a leading part. The rash appears to be a bodily eruption from the inside out and it doesn't make sense to treat it only with topical creams designed to suppress the itch, important though symptom relief is. Herbalists examine the diet carefully and may try careful food-elimination tests to identify culprits.

Milk is a common factor in childhood eczema. Excess nervous tension can exacerbate eczema, and cooling or relaxing remedies are often indicated. The elimination systems are important so blood, liver, bowels and kidneys are given attention.

Charlie was put on a milk-free diet for two weeks. This requires cutting out milk on breakfast cereal, butter, cheese, yoghurts, warm school milk, and all those milk puddings. I asked his mother to check carefully all packaged food because of the large number that contain some form of milk, especially skimmed milk. It is usually hidden in the ingredients list as whey, skim milk, SMP (skimmed milk powder), or dairy solids.

Charlie and his mother were both encouraged to eat less fried food and more fresh vegetables and fruits. I managed to encourage them to go for chicken instead of sausages and fish fingers.

The herbal treatment aimed to stimulate lymphatic emptying, elimination processes in the liver and digestive tract, and mildly stimulate of the body's own source of steroids, the adrenal glands.

HERBAL PRESCRIPTION

Two remedies were given. First was a light cream of chickweed *(Stellllria media)* and marigold *(Calendula officinolis)* 50:50 to relieve the itch and keep the eczema moist to reduce cracking and weeping. The second was a tincture:

HERBAL PRESCRIPTION		
Burdock	*Arctium lappa*	15 ml
Heartsease	*Viola tricolor*	20 ml
Dandelion root	*Taraxacum rfficinale*	20 ml
Liquorice	*radix*	10 ml
Figwort	*Glycyrrhiza glabra*	10 ml
Verbena	*Scrophularia nodosa*	25 ml
	Verbena officinolis	100 ml
Dose: 3 ml, three times daily in water before meals.		

The cream eased the itch, making Charlie's life tolerable. It reduced his irritability and improved his ability to concentrate at school. He now sleeps at night.
The tincture helped calm the rash which became less angry and was less likely to crack and weep. After one month it began to fade to a light superficial redness with little itching. His digestion and general appearance improved and he became more relaxed and happy.
Cutting out milk seemed to reduce the eczema dramatically, this was tested after two weeks by adding milk back into the diet and the rash became worse, although not as bad as it was originally.

After 6 months, the diet alone seems to be controlling the rash. Milk has been reduced by more than 75 per cent. It is very difficult to eliminate completely, and this is not usually necessary. The family have improved their diet dramatically. It is far from perfect but is so much better than when they first came that they feel they have struck a significant blow for their own family health and swear they all feel better for it.

Acne and Hair Loss

Samantha was a 19-year-old student in Cambridge. She came with recurrent spots which were worse during her period. There were occasional rashes around her mouth and she regularly had vaginal thrush. She also had falling hair which came out 'in handfuls' as she brushed her hair and she felt itchy all over her body most of the time. The history showed a rundown metabolism, drained from excessive student lifestyle, and suggested an impaired immune system. Samantha drank alcohol nightly and often partied until the early hours during the week. She smoked marijuana daily and took a cocktail 'of other fashionable drugs, including ecstasy, ephedrine and 'magic mushrooms '. Her diet was inadequate, consisting of coffee, take-away pizzas and curries, and pub meals.
Examination showed a normal liver but some tenderness over the gall bladder suggesting inflammation, an otherwise normal abdomen, no signs of infection on the scalp or elsewhere on the skin. There were no signs of jaundice. Cursory signs of anaemia were absent but a full blood test was advised.
Samantha had otherwise been reasonably healthy throughout her life until two years previously. After a period of 10 months' international travel, followed by a move from a university in Bristol to Cambridge University, the problems started and accumulated.

This seemed like a patient with possible mild hepatitis from excess alcohol and other drugs. Liver function may have been significantly reduced without serious damage to the liver being evident. The lifestyle and poor diet would not have done much for her immune system, which may also have been suppressed.

HERBAL APPROACH

Treatment began with negotiating a commitment to cut all drugs and to reduce alcohol to one or two nights a week, without any drunkenness. To my surprise she was sufficiently shocked by her condition to agree to try this drastic change to lifestyle.
A new diet was discussed, with more reliance on fruits and vegetables with pulse dishes and less of the take-away and high fat
pub meal type dishes. Fewer nights out in the pub meant more money and time for preparing better food at home. Herbal treatment was directed at supporting the liver, cleansing the blood and boosting the immune system. A hair rinse was given to stimulate circulation to the scalp.

HERBAL PRESCRIPTION		
Echinacea	*Echinacea angustifolia*	40 ml
Fumitory	*Fumaria officinalis*	20 ml
Barberry	*Berberis vulgaris*	20 ml
'Milk thistle	*Cardus marianus*	20 ml
Chilli	*Capsicum minimum*	1 ml
		101 ml
Dose: 5 ml three times daily before food.		

In addition a herbal tea was given. It was equal parts of:

Marigold	*Calendula officina/is*
Rosemary	*Rosmarinus officina/is*
Dandelion leaf	*Taraxacum officinale folia*
Heartsease	*Viola tricolor*

The tea was prepared with 1 teaspoon of the mixed herbs
and one mugful was taken three times daily.
Over three months, her skin progressively cleared up, and
the hair loss stopped. The facial rashes and thrush
disappeared, and she began feeling much more energetic and
generally healthy.
Twelve months on she had managed to stick to the low
alcohol better lifestyle contract and her health has been
maintained.

Piles (Haemorrhoids)

John, a 45-year-old bus driver, came with itching around the
anus and constipation. The history also found that he often
passed small amounts of blood streaked on his stools or
showing bright red on the lavatory paper. His bowel
movements were infrequent (only every 3 or 4 days) and the
motions were often difficult to pass. He often suffered from
pains in the left side of the abdomen and these were relieved
by opening his bowels. For John, these were normal bowel
movements, for he had known nothing different. He
suffered from headaches, colic and discomfort. in the
abdomen.
His diet consisted of white sliced bread toast in the morning,
pies or sausages with chips for lunch, and hamburgers with
mashed potato or fish and chips for supper. He ate only two
or three pieces of fruit a week and snacked on confectionery
bars or biscuits for his coffee breaks on the driving shift.
The low fiber content of this diet could cause the
constipation which, together with his sedentary job, may
explain the piles.

Abdominal examination was normal. Examination of the back passage showed swollen inflamed veins and one prolapsed vein or haemorrhoid. There was a small anal fissure which was red and weeping slightly. Both the haemorrhoid and the fissure could have explained the itching.

HERBAL APPROACH

Treatment consisted of attending to the state of the digestive system to get a better flow through the intestines and to ensure that the stools were soft and easy to pass without overstretching the anus or requiring much muscle straining to pass them out.

This is best done with diet but to start the process moving and get early relief of symptoms, the patient was given flea seed husks (1 dessertspoon, twice a day in water) to provide a large and soft stool. The diet was changed to wholemeal bread, a breakfast of high-cereal muesli, with two pieces of fruit daily.

For snacks, John ate 5-10 dried apricots a day and fresh fruit or a carrot instead of confectionery. The diet was monitored to see how successfully he could change and sustain the higher fibre diet. Only in the event of hardship or failure were daily doses of bran to be considered. They weren't needed.

HERBAL TREATMENT

Herbs were directed first to maintain a healthy liver and bile activity, both of which encourage more efficient bowel activity and support the dietary change:

HERBAL PRESCRIPTION		
Barberry	*Berberis vulgaris*	10 ml
Dandelion root *officinale*	*Taraxacum officinale*	30 ml
radix	*radix*	30 ml
Yellow dock	*Rumex crispus*	30 ml
Horse chestnut	*Aesculus hippoeaslanum*	100 ml
Dose: 5 ml three times daily before food.		

In addition, suppositories of horse chestnut and tormentil *(Potentilla ereela)* were prepared using a cocoa butter base. These were inserted twice daily, morning and night *after* bowel movements to tone and heal the haemorrhoids. After three days his bowel motions became looser and more frequent. After a week there was little straining. In fact, his motions became so thin that the stool was ribbon-like rather than his normal round pellets. I reassured him that the ribbon type was what everybody should be aiming for. The itch stopped in two weeks along with the spotting and streaking of blood. He has had no troubles since and has maintained his healthier diet.

ME (Myalgic Encephalomyelitis)/Post-Viral Fatigue Syndrome

Marella was a 33-year-old Swiss woman who presented with fears of anaemia. She had had painful periods and was totally listless, without energy. These symptoms had persisted for nearly two years and had not been experienced before. She found her job in theatrical management difficult as by lunchtime each day she wanted only to sleep. The job was stressful but her personal life was relaxed and happy. She used to be physically active, swimming regularly, but could no longer cope with exercise. Any exercise usually meant she needed three days to recover tolerable energy levels, which were rapidly depleted.

I had her do a full blood test and this was totally normal with the exception of a slight rise in one type of white blood cell, suggesting she may have had a recent allergic reaction. There was no sign of anaemia or other abnormality to explain the listlessness. She had no tenderness in her muscles or aching after exercise.

Her history brought out that she had been very ill with chicken pox two years ago and that she had never felt really herself since. Closer questioning suggested that the symptoms stemmed from this illness. She had also been given no less than five courses of antibiotics over the previous two years after dental work for an abscess. Marella also had symptoms of an irritable bowel with bloating, irregularity and alternating diarrhoea and constipation. She had been experiencing bad period pain and worsening PMT for at least eight days before the flow began.

HERBAL APPROACH

This looked like an example of what I prefer to call post-viral syndrome. There was no muscle weakness and tenderness, which is often reported in ME, but the whole condition is such a mixture of varying symptoms that there can be no typical case.

There were other signs of battered immune and metabolic systems with her irritable bowel and disturbed menstrual cycle.

Treatment was aimed at stimulating her immune system against a persistent virus clinging on in her nerve tissue, and at boosting her entire bodily system to lift it above the depressant effect of the previous infection.

HERBAL PRESCRIPTION

My approach in this case was clear and simple. Echinacea to boost her immune system coupled with Siberian ginseng, which is an efficient adaptogen that stimulates the functioning of the body's systems and general metabolism.

HERBAL PRESCRIPTION		
Elutherococcus	*Elutherococcus senticosus*	50 ml
Echinacea		40 ml
Dandelion root	*Echinacea angustifolia*	10 ml
	Taraxacum tfficinale radix	100 ml
Dose: 5 ml four times daily for one week then three times daily.		

After one week, Marella realized how much her after-work energy was restored when she found herself cleaning her flat late in the evening when she would normally have been sleeping.

Over the following six weeks her energy improved consistently to the extent that she is now exercising gently, is not listless after work and her digestive symptoms have reduced considerably.

Chest Infections/Colds

Robert was 21 and felt hard done by. He seemed to have three or four colds every year and during the winter months seemed to be with a constant cold. His colds started suddenly with a sore throat, progressed rapidly through various stuffy stages with yellow to green catarrh and often took two or even three weeks to clear. He was left with constant catarrh and occasional sinusitis. He felt run down, low in energy and concentration.

The history brought out a general tendency to infections. He had occasional boils and had had two attacks of what sounded like cystitis in the past year. He had athlete's foot on the right foot and this had come and gone for the last three years. Robert used to be healthier but since he left home and started living in Birmingham, where he worked as a clerk, his health had slipped. He had little exercise and his diet was based on convenience foods at home and hamburgers on nights 'out with the boys'. He smoked 25 cigarettes daily.

HERBAL APPROACH

Anyone can get a cold each winter, but repeated infections are a sign of a lowered immune response. Healthy bodies encourage healthy immune systems to protect them. It is as though neglected bodies don't see any point in wasting energy maintaining their immune system.

Robert's diet and lifestyle left much room for improvement. Healthy eating is essential to maintain adequate nutrition to fight infections. Exercise and relaxation also help to optimize functioning of all systems. We agreed a deal where if I could show him fewer colds in six months, he would go the whole way and quit smoking. A new flat mate who was interested in cooking made the essential dietary changes possible and practical. More fruit and veg with less stodgy and convenience foods were the plan. A session on cooking tips and a list of starter cookery books from the library provided motivation and the means to change.

Exercise started as cycling to work but he now plays squash at his work social club.

Herbal treatment concentrated on cleansing his system, stimulating it and encouraging the immune response. The tincture was started as he began the dietary and exercise changes. He was encouraged to take a starter dose of 100 mg vitamin C every day for the next three months and to do so during the winter months as a matter of course.

HERBAL PRESCRIPTION		
Echinacea	*Echinacea angustifolia*	45 ml
Marigold	*Calendula officinalis*	20 ml
Damiana	*Turnera diffusa*	30 ml
Wormwood	*Artemisia absinthium*	5 ml
		100 ml
Dose: 5 ml three times daily before meals.		

After four weeks there was improvement in his upper respiratory symptoms. After another four weeks he was much better; he was taken off the tincture and given a maintenance tea of equal parts marigold and rosemary to be taken three times daily. He continued to improve. The cystitis has not reappeared after 12 months and the sinusitis has gone and not reappeared.

His next winter's colds numbered only two and he has respected his part of the bargain and given up cigarettes, but not without a struggle. .

Anxiety/Insomnia

Mary, 52 years old, arrived at the clinic asking for 'something to help me sleep'. She said she hadn't slept well for three weeks.

Her husband had been made redundant twice in the past year and, because of his age, they were worried about his chances of future employment. Mary managed the family budget and she was in fear of losing their house and having to cancel the family holiday, and worse.

In discussion, we decided that simple worry was keeping her from sleeping well. She would drop off easily around 11 pm but would wake promptly at 3 am and toss and turn, unable to get back to sleep. She was waking exhausted and unable to cope with her day. She was also eating badly, skipping meals because of loss of appetite and was smoking more than before. To help her sleep she had begun drinking alcohol before bed but had not found it helped. She was becoming constipated.

Her husband was depressed and both were getting more irritable and unable to talk without snapping.

HERBAL APPROACH

Anxiety is a terrible burden. It can take over our lives quickly. Mary's disturbed sleep pattern is typical of anxiety sufferers and makes the anxiety worse because tiredness makes it more difficult to cope with the problems that are causing the sleep problem. Matters usually get worse and worse. Sleep is desperately sought but is only very short-term relief unless the cause of the anxiety can be tackled. Anxiety, and stress in general, also cause physical problems like ulcers, constipation and irritable bowel so are worth tackling quickly in the interest of health.

There are herbal hypnotics, which induce sleep efficiently, but I use these as a last resort. Far better to try to help with the cause of the anxiety and to support with herbal remedies that relieve the anxiety. These help clear any panicked thought about the problems and allow a healthier sleep without sedation.

For Mary, we plotted new avenues for finding work for her husband. He had been a builder's merchant so his knowledge of the trade after 34 years' work was worth turning into a consultant's business. He was interested and started a local course in small business management on a grant. This got him motivated, and soon after spreading the word among his previous contacts, he had offers of work. Mary's insomnia was tackled with the initial help of calming herbs and support to her stressed nervous system. Getting involved in motivating her husband diverted her worry to the positive anxiety of the challenge. With the herbs she was more able to cope, slept better and her physical symptoms receded.

HERBAL PRESCRIPTION

She did not need knock-out herbs to force sleep but gentle anxiolytics to reduce anxiety reaction and to calm.

HERBAL PRESCRIPTION		
Skullcap	*Scutdlaria latenfolia*	50 ml
Vervain	*Verbena officina/is*	30 ml
Dandelion root	*Taraxacum officinale*	15 ml
Gentian	*radix*	5 ml
	Gentiana lutea	100 ml
Dose: 5 ml four times daily for two weeks.		

In addition Mary was encouraged to take a warm bath each evening and to drop five drops of lavender oil into the water after she lowered herself in. This relaxes body and mind and encourages a restful sleep. '

After two weeks Mary found the herbs had allowed her to sleep and feel much calmer. She then took the tincture only as needed, usually at 10ml before bed. It took five months for her husband to get on to the course but over those months they both were working together towards a goal that could solve the initial problems. As far as I know he is satisfied in his new work, Mary has become a business partner and has learned to tackle her anxiety and sleeps soundly.

Menopausal Symptoms

Many women prefer to avoid HRT (hormone replacement therapy) but still want to avoid the unpleasant side effects of menopause. Joan found her periods stopped suddenly two years before she came to see me. She was 54 when the sudden change occurred and experienced severe hot flushes, tachycardia (rapid heartbeats), and dizziness. She had a responsible job as a nurse and needed to reduce the symptoms so she could keep working. She tried HRT but could stand it only for eight months because of the side effects of headaches, nausea, water retention and rashes. The consultation showed she was still having hot flushes and headaches as well as feeling giddy much of the day. She was suffering from stress from pressure at work and several longstanding family problems. She also had been experiencing a burning sensation on her lips and inner cheeks, which added to her stress. Her bowels were erratic and she was not sleeping well, often waking two or three times in a night.

HERBAL APPROACH

Herbalists see the menopause as a normal process that should not be delayed by supplying the oestrogen that the ovaries have stopped providing. The strategy is to calm the body's responses to natural oestrogen withdrawal and to help reduce any tendency to overexcite the nervous system. In short, the body is cooled or calmed.

HERBAL PRESCRIPTION

A tincture of:

HERBAL PRESCRIPTION		
Hawthorn	*Crataegus oxycanthvides*	20 ml
Motherwort	*Leonurus cardiaca*	30 ml
Lady's mantle	*Alchemilit] vulgaris*	20 ml
Helonias root	*Chamaelirium luteum*	20 ml
Vitex	*Vitex agnus-castus*	10 ml
		100 ml
Dose: 5 ml three times daily.		

After two weeks there were fewer hot flushes, especially in the day and less sign of palpitation. Stress was still evident and seemed to be dominating her life and she was clearly agitated. I included a second tincture aimed at helping her cope with the stress of the domestic problems.

HERBAL PRESCRIPTION		
Skullcap	*Scutellaria laterifolia*	50 ml
Betony	*Stachys betonica*	25 ml
St John's Wort	*Hypericum perforatum*	25 ml
		100 ml
Dose: 5 ml three times daily before food.		

After four weeks the flushes, headaches and heart symptoms had all but gone. Occasional flushes appeared but they were very mild and no longer bothered Joan. The burning lips were unrelated to the menopausal symptoms, but were eventually cured: we discovered that Joan's new top denture plate was *3/16th* inch too high between the top lip and the gums, pressing on a nerve and causing the uncomfortable symptoms. Using her old dentures solved the problem while the dentist adjusted the new set. The problem has not reappeared. It is very common for dental work, especially root canal or molar extractions, to initiate nerve irritation around the mouth.

Chapter Eight

Home Remedies

Using herbal remedies at home recreates the history of herbal medicine. It also provides safe, efficient and cheap medicines.

Not only were herbs often the only available medicines but they were, and continue to be, medicinal plants growing around every village and town as well as in the countryside. The Bible chronicles the tradition and authority for this belief in Psalms 104, 'He causeth herbs to grow for the service of man.' Each household either knew where useful herbs could be harvested when needed or had a store of dried material and prepared medicaments ready for use.

A basic home-remedy kit can be prepared for modern use. My personal approach is based on the following criteria:

• a small number of effective herbs, which are
• safe to use,
• simple to prepare and administer,
• cover the main common ailments, and
• can be found in most kitchens, gardens, local parks or commons.

The herbs I have chosen are very safe to use. When used as recommended there is no reason to believe they can cause harm.

Using home remedies is safe if simple rules are followed. After all, we treat ourselves regularly whenever we buy cough sweets, vitamin supplements, or aspirin. The rules are important because they mean we are more likely to be successful with home remedies as well as safer.

Treat only conditions where the diagnosis is obvious.

Conditions like colds, bee stings, travel sickness, bruises and scalds are unlikely to be confused with anything more serious. But if in any doubt with the diagnosis, make sure you see a qualified herbalist or your doctor before you embark on a course of self-treatment. Making the wrong diagnosis by yourself might mean choosing the wrong remedy and thus having no healing benefit. But far worse is the risk that you might misdiagnose, or not even notice signs of a serious illness. Confirming the diagnosis doesn't mean you cannot treat yourself, it means you know what you are trying to treat. I recommend you take heed of the home-herbalist's charter:

Whenever in doubt about the diagnosis or the right treatment *always check;* any diarrhoea, pain in the abdomen, chest or head, or any dizzy spells or fainting that last more than three days should be reported to a qualified herbalist or your doctor, even if you think you know the cause.

The home remedy kit lists 24 herbs which could form the basic starter kit. Note that most herbs have several different actions which make them useful for more than one type of condition.

All are simple to use and easy to harvest or to buy. The list of conditions suggests which herb or herbs can be used. Sometimes more than one herb is suggested.

Herbs For The Home Remedy Kit

Herb	Conditions	Form Used
Arnica	bruises, sprains	tincture, cream
Calendula	cuts, stings, rashes, burns, thrush, athlete's foot	tincture, infusion, cream
Chamomile	digestion, rashes, burns, restlessness, teething	infusion, cream
Clove oil	toothache	oil
Comfrey	sprains, wounds, psoriasis	fresh leaf poultice, cream
Dandelion	water retention, digestion, warts	infusion, sap (warts)
Elder flower	Hay fever, catarrh, colds, flu	infusion
Eucalyptus	wounds, colds, flu, sinusitis	oil, inhalation
Fennel	digestion, flatulence, colic	seeds, infusion
Feverfew	migraine, rheumatic pain	fresh or dried leaf, tincture
Figs	mild laxative	fruit, syrup
Garlic	antiseptic, catarrh, lung infections, food poisoning, worms, warts	whole cloves, pearls, tablets
Ginger	chilblains, cold hands and feet, travel sickness,	fresh or powdered root

	morning sickness	
Lavender	antiseptic, wounds, stings, bites, muscle spasm, relaxant	oil
Lemon balm	restlessness, insomnia	fresh or frozen herb infusion
Lime flower	flu, fevers, relaxant, restless children, insomnia	infusion
Marshmallow	boils, splinters, sore throats, oesophagitis	infusion, poultice
Mint	digestion, flatulence, colic	infusion
Myrrh	cuts, wounds; mouth wash for sore throats and mouth ulcers	tincture
Oak bark (powder)	bleeding or weeping wounds, mouth ulcers, gingivitis	infusion, powder
Ribwort	bleeding wounds, sore throats, catarrh	infusion
St John's Wort	burns, earache, sciatica, wounds, menstrual pain	infusion, infused oil
Thyme	colds, congested chests, respiratory infections, worms	tincture, infusion
Yarrow	nosebleeds, fever management	bruised leaf, infusion

There are no 'one and only' remedies for most common ailments but the following table lists tried and trusted remedies that are easy to apply and safe to use.

Ailments and Helpful Home Remedies

Ailment	Home Remedies
Antiseptic	Washes with infusions of calendula, lotions of myrrh or lavender oil diluted in water, or cut fresh garlic rubbed onto the affected part. Fresh garlic disinfects the stomach.
Bites/stings	Dab lavender oil or calendula tincture on neat.
Boils/spots	A poultice of marshmallow will draw out a boil and neat oil of lavender or tincture of calendula helps heal and protect.
Bleeding grazes or wounds	Sprinkling of oak bark or applying a poultice of ribwort leaf helps stop bleeding. Calendula tincture and lavender or eucalyptus oil will keep germ-free.

Bruises/ sprams	Arnica or comfrey cream applied regularly, or wrap a freshly crushed comfrey leaf around the part daily.
Burns	First degree burns where the skin is red and slightly blistered heal with St John's Wort infused oil or washing with infusions of calendula or chamomile. Let dry or wrap in crushed fresh comfrey leaf.
Catarrh	Infusions of elder flower and ribwort if catarrh is not infected; otherwise include thyme and eat garlic.
Chilblains	Ginger root infusion warms the peripheral areas.

Colds	Eat garlic or drink thyme infusions to kill bacteria; take elder flower and lime flower teas to manage the fever which helps kill the virus. (See sore throats.)
Cold sores	Apply neat lavender or lemon balm oil, or tincture of calendula.
Colic	See digestion. Children's and babies' colic can be relieved with half strength chamomile or peppermint tea.
Diarrhoea	Treat only mild diarrheas. Use garlic or thyme if due to food poisoning, and strong black tea of decoctions of oak bark to stop the diarrhea.
Digestion (poor or sluggish)	Dandelion root infusion or leaf as salad to stimulate but infusions of chamomile, mint, ginger, or fennel to calm.

Earache/ear boils	Infused oil of St John's wort, 3-4 drops twice daily.
Fevers (mild)	Controlled, not stopped, with infusions of elder flower and lime flower.
Flatulence	Fennel seeds chewed; infusions of chamomile, mint or ginger.
Flu	See colds.
Food poising	Mild forms solved by eating 3-5 cloves garlic daily or infusion of thyme.
Gingivitis	Oak bark powder made into thin paste as mouthwash or myrrh tincture diluted 1:10 with water as mouthwash.
Hay fever	Start two months before season with elder flower and ribwort infusion daily.
Headache	Migraines often stopped or prevented with 3-5 fresh or dried leaves of feverfew daily; nervous headache eased by relaxing with lemon balm or lime flower infusions.

Insomnia	The cause must be found, but mild anxious forms eased with lime flower or lemon balm infusions before bed and no caffeine drinks after midday. Sitting in a warm bath with 5-10 drops of lavender oil before bed is very successful.
Morning sickness	Infusion of chamomile, ginger or mint.
Mouth ulcers	Tincture of myrrh applied neat or used as a mouthwash diluted 1:10in water.
Muscle spasms	Lavender oil, 1 teaspoon in an egg cup of household vegetable oil and gently massaged into the affected parts. Carefully insert a bruised
Nosebleeds	Carefully insert a bruised leaf of yarrow into the bleeding nostril with the leaf protruding. Pinch nostrils together for 10 minutes.
Piles	Cream of oak bark and marigold.

Psoriasis	Comfrey and marigold cream.
Rashes	Infusions or compresses of chamomile or marigold for irritations like eczema, seborrhoea, nappy rash; marigold tincture neat on fungal rashes.
Respiratory infections	Thyme infusions or garlic cloves. See sore throats.
Restless children	Infusion of lime flower or chamomile.
Relaxation	Infusion of lemon balm, lime flower or chamomile.
Rheumatic pain	Feverfew as fresh leaf or tincture for pain; dandelion root decoction to help elimination processes.
Sinusitis	Steam inhalation with thyme and eucalyptus oils.
Sore throats	Gargle with one part myrrh tincture diluted in 10 of water; painful throat soothed with sipping strong infusion of marshmallow.

Splinters	A poultice of marshmallow leaf will draw them out.
Thrush	Infusion or tincture of marigold as wash on body and as douche for vaginal thrush.
Travel sickness	Chew 1/8th inch slice fresh ginger root 20 minutes before travel and then during travel.
Teething pain	Infusion of chamomile.
Toothache	One of two drops of clove oil on the culprit.
Warts	Apply fresh dandelion latex - the white sap from the leaves and roots - or garlic juice daily for 2-3 weeks.
Water retention	Infusion of dandelion leaf.
Worms	Infusion of thyme or fresh garlic cloves.

Preparations

Herbalists use a wide range of preparations to deliver their medicines to the affected parts. The most common are tinctures and infusions, which are extracts of herbs in alcohol or water respectively. Creams and ointments are also used regularly to place medications on or under the skin. But pills, tablets, powders, pessaries, suppositories, lotions, linctuses, syrups, compresses and poultices are also widely used. Most of these are fiddly to make at home but are rarely essential for effective treatment. The simple preparations recommended in the ailments list above are excellent for home remedies.

INFUSIONS

A cup of tea is an infusion. Herbal infusions are also made with water but should be allowed to stand for 10-15minutes, the longer the better. They are used to extract water-soluble components of plants like mucilage, tannins, saponins and flavonoids. They do not extract fixed oils or much alkaloid, which require a mixture of alcohol and water to dissolve them.

Herbal infusions are made with 1 oz (30 g) herb to 1 pint of boiling water. Always use a teapot with a good lid or a thermos flask to keep the volatile oils from being lost. The usual dosage for adults is one cup or small mug three times a day. Wait for it to cool first if you wish. For children older than 10 years, use half the adult dose (V2 oz in 1 pint water) and for infants (3-10) use a quarter.

DECOCTIONS

Tough plant material like roots and bark needs more vigorous extraction than a simple infusion. A decoction is made from plant material boiled gently in water for 15 minutes. The resulting extract is strained and used like an infusion.

CREAMS

Creams are useful for applying medicine to affected skin. Sometimes the medicine is needed on the skin (as in eczema), or cream is used so the medication can be absorbed through to skin to reach affected parts like joints. Creams are also soothing to the skin.

Marigold/calendula cream (herbal as well as homoeopathic) can be bought but it is easy to make your own. The simplest way is to use emulsifying ointment BP, which can be bought in good chemists. Make a double strength infusion of chosen herb or a mixture (for example chamomile, marigold or comfrey).

Take 50 g of ointment and heat it gently in a double boiler (or over a water bath) until it melts. Add'25 ml of the infusion. Take the mixture from the heat and stir gently until it starts to thicken. Add five drops of friar's balsam (to preserve the cream).

Pour or spoon the cream into small jars and seal. *Label straight away before you forget th£, herb used, and date the batch.* Use small amounts of emulsifying ointment, unless you have an army to treat. A little cream goes a long way and lasts a long time (12 months in a cool, dark place).

INFUSED OIL

An infused oil is a way of extracting the medicinal value of a herb into an oil which can then be applied directly to the skin or used to make thicker ointments. St John's Wort oil is simple to make. Harvest enough of the yellow flowers during the summer to fill a 1 or 2 lb screw-cap jam jar. Pour over the fresh flowers enough sunflower or maize (corn) oil to fill the jar. Place the jar in a sunny spot for 4-6 weeks. The oil turns a deep red and the constituents of the flowers diffuse out into the oil.

Decant the oil into a clean dark jar for use. Infused oils of other plants, like comfrey, can be made by heating chopped herb in the oil over a water bath for six hours, then pressing out the oil and filtering it.

POULTICE

This is a useful way of applying herbs to the skin. They are usually applied hot, which increases the blood flow to the area and encourages uptake of the herbs as well as healing action.

A poultice of marshmallow is useful on boils or splinters. Take 1 dessertspoon of dried herb and moisten with boiling water. When cooled to a tolerable temperature, place over the boil or splinter and hold in place by tying a muslin bandage over the herb. Leave for one hour then repeat.

Drying Herbs

Many of the herbs in the home remedy kit grow in gardens, parks or where relaxing country walks can be organized. Harvesting and drying herbs preserves their medicinal value and means they are always available. A few simple rules will help you have the best quality herbs.

• Always make sure you know which species of plant is used and that you can identify it.

• Harvest the right part/s of the plant and harvest them at the best time of year. Most leaves and flowering parts are best during the flowering period. Roots and barks are best harvested in the autumn.

• Dry the herbs carefully by spreading them out in a thin layer on paper in a warm (not hot), well-aerated room, which is protected from full sun. Roots should be washed and cut into 4 inch pieces before they are dried.

• When dried, herbs should be stored in paper bags in a dry, dark room.

• Make sure every herb is carefully labeled with name and harvest date. It is remarkable how similar many plants look when they are dried.

EXPAND YOUR HERB COLLECTION

There are many other herbs that are useful for home remedies. As you gain confidence and skill, try other plants recommended for the ailments listed here. Take care to read about the plant and its uses before you embark on experimentation. A list of useful books and other sources of additional information is found in chapter 11.

www.ingramcontent.com/pod-product-compliance
Lightning Source LLC
Chambersburg PA
CBHW070356290526
45790CB00004B/1513